ECHO
MADE EASY

This book is dedicated to my parents.

ECHO
MADE EASY

Third Edition

Sam Kaddoura
BSc(Hons), BM BCh(Oxon), PhD, DIC, FRCP, FESC, FACC

Consultant Cardiologist
Chelsea and Westminster Hospital and
Royal Brompton Hospital, London, UK

Honorary Consultant Cardiologist
Royal Hospital Chelsea, London, UK

Honorary Senior Lecturer
Imperial College School of Medicine, London, UK

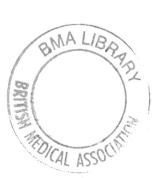

ELSEVIER

Edinburgh   London   New York   Oxford   Philadelphia   St Louis   Sydney   Toronto 2016

ELSEVIER

First edition 2002
Second edition 2009
Third edition 2016

Classical Chinese editions 2003 and 2010
Turkish edition 2005
Simplified Chinese edition 2006
Korean edition 2008
Polish edition 2008
Spanish edition 2010
Portuguese edition 2010

Notices

Knowledge and best practice in this field are constantly changing. As new research and experience broaden our understanding, changes in research methods, professional practices, or medical treatment may become necessary.

Practitioners and researchers must always rely on their own experience and knowledge in evaluating and using any information, methods, compounds, or experiments described herein. In using such information or methods they should be mindful of their own safety and the safety of others, including parties for whom they have a professional responsibility.

With respect to any drug or pharmaceutical products identified, readers are advised to check the most current information provided (i) on procedures featured or (ii) by the manufacturer of each product to be administered, to verify the recommended dose or formula, the method and duration of administration, and contraindications. It is the responsibility of practitioners, relying on their own experience and knowledge of their patients, to make diagnoses, to determine dosages and the best treatment for each individual patient, and to take all appropriate safety precautions.

To the fullest extent of the law, neither the Publisher nor the authors, contributors, or editors, assume any liability for any injury and/or damage to persons or property as a matter of products liability, negligence or otherwise, or from any use or operation of any methods, products, instructions, or ideas contained in the material herein.

ISBN 978-0-7020-6656-6
[International Edition ISBN 978-0-7020-6657-3]

Printed in China
Last digit is the print number: 9 8 7 6 5 4 3

Senior Content Strategist: **Laurence Hunter**
Senior Content Development Specialist: **Ailsa Laing**
Senior Project Manager: **Beula Christopher**
Design: **Christian Bilbow**
Illustration Manager: **Karen Giacomucci**
Illustrator: **Robert Britton**

Working together
to grow libraries in
developing countries

www.elsevier.com • www.bookaid.org

CONTENTS

5 Transoesophageal, 3-D and Stress Echo and Other Echo Techniques

6 Cardiac Masses, Infection, Congenital Abnormalities and Aorta

7 Special Situations and Conditions

8 Performing and Reporting an Echo

PREFACE

Echocardiography (echo) is the use of ultrasound to examine the heart. It is a powerful and safe technique which has become widely available for cardiovascular investigation. The training of medical students and newly qualified doctors often includes an introduction to echo. Undergraduate and postgraduate examinations such as MRCP (UK) sometimes set questions on the subject.

While there are many detailed texts of echo available, aimed primarily at cardiologists and those performing echo examinations, such as cardiac physiologists, there are few simply introductory texts.

This book aims to provide a practical and clinically useful introduction to echo – much of which *is* easy – for those who will be using, requesting and possibly performing and interpreting it in the future. The book is aimed particularly at doctors in training and medical students. It is also hoped that it may be of interest to other groups – established physicians, surgeons and general practitioners, cardiac physiologists and cardiac technicians, nurses and paramedics. There are national and international accreditation programmes and examinations in echo, and this may be a starting introductory book for those hoping ultimately to gain echo training and certification.

It aims to explain the echo techniques available, what an echo can and cannot give, and – importantly – puts echo into a clinical perspective. It is by no means intended as a complete textbook of echo, and some aspects are far beyond its scope (e.g. complex congenital heart disease and paediatric echo).

Since publication of the first edition in 2002 and the second edition in 2009, *Echo Made Easy* has been translated from English into seven languages; Standard Mandarin and simplified Chinese, Spanish, Portuguese, Korean, Turkish and Polish.

This new, third edition has become necessary because of advances in echocardiography over the past 6 years. The book has been updated throughout. A new chapter – Performing and Reporting an Echo – has been added. New sections include the role of echo in individuals with cancer and in diseases of the aorta. There are updated and expanded sections on pregnancy, the continuity equation, diastolic function, long-axis function and 3-D echo. There are also updates and more detailed sections on the use of echo in emergency situations, in cardiomyopathies and pericardial diseases, in congenital abnormalities and in cardiac resynchronization therapy. Up-to-date published international guidelines have been referenced throughout.

New online content is available (echo video images, data interpretation and multiple choice questions [MCQs]) and this has two main objectives: to allow the reader to carry out self-assessment of knowledge (for example, if preparing for accreditation examinations) and to see examples of echos described in the text.

The intention has been to keep the book around the same length as the previous edition, but inevitably there has been some increase due to new figures and text. There has been a small increase in page size, allowing for larger images, but the book should remain compact. Full colour illustrations are used throughout for this new edition.

Sam Kaddoura
London
2016

ACKNOWLEDGEMENTS

I am very grateful to Professor A. R. Kaddoura and Dr N. Shamaa for their enormous help in the preparation of the book. A number of individuals have made helpful contributions to this third edition or to previous editions. I should like to thank Dr Victoria Simpkin, Dr Ali Vizir, Dr Farhan Abdul Hamid, Mrs Sonia Williams, Miss Valentina Santamaria, Mrs Fatima Cortez, Miss Raquel Nunes and Mr Darren White. My thanks also to Dr Derek Gibson, Miss Fiona Trent, Mr Roel Caneja, Dr Sabine Ernst, Dr Jan Till, Dr Pavandeep Ghataorhe, Dr Michael Pelly, Dr Abbas Khakoo, Professor Mark Johnson, Dr Kenric Li, Dr George Buyanovsky, Professor Michael Gatzoulis, Dr Lorna Swan, Miss Roshni Patel, Professor John Pepper, Dr Jonathan Clague, Dr Ed Leatham and Dr Julian Collinson. Thanks to Kate Pool and the Society of Authors, Dr Phil Carrillo, Dr Gerry Carr-White, Dr Michael Henein, Dr Rohan Jagathesan, Mrs Johan Carberry, Mrs Myrle Crathern, Mrs Renomee Porten, Dr Sanjay Prasad, Mrs Denise Udo and Dr Ihab Ramzy. I am also grateful to Mrs Natalie Martin, Professor Jamil Mayet, Dr Rakesh Sharma, Dr Wei Li, Miss Beth Unsworth and Mr Graham Clark. Last but not least, many thanks to the team at Churchill Livingstone Elsevier for their kind help and advice: especially Ms Ailsa Laing, Mrs Beula Christopher, Mrs Janice Urquhart, Ms Christine Johnston and Susan Jansons. Thanks also to Mr Robert Britton. The idea for *Echo Made Easy* followed a meeting with Mr Laurence Hunter some years ago. I remain grateful to Laurence for his continued support and friendship.

Sam Kaddoura
London
2016

ABBREVIATIONS

2-D	Two-dimensional
3-D	Three-dimensional
5-HT	5-Hydroxytryptamine
A$_2$	Aortic second heart sound
A$_m$ (or a′, A′)	Atrial myocardial velocity
A2C	Apical 2-chamber
A3C	Apical 3-chamber
A4C	Apical 4-chamber
A5C	Apical 5-chamber
A-wave	Atrial wave of mitral flow
AC	Arrhythmogenic cardiomyopathy
ACC	American College of Cardiology
ACE	Angiotensin-converting enzyme
AF	Atrial fibrillation
AHA	American Heart Association
AMVL	Anterior mitral valve leaflet
Ao	Aorta
AR	Aortic regurgitation
ARVC	Arrhythmogenic right ventricular cardiomyopathy
ARVD	Arrhythmogenic right ventricular dysplasia
AS	Aortic stenosis
ASD	Atrial septal defect
ASE	Americal Society of Echocardiography
ASH	Asymmetrical septal hypertrophy
AT	Acceleration time
AV	Aortic valve
BART	Blue away, red towards
BP	Blood pressure
BSA	Body surface area
BSE	British Society of Echocardiography
CABG	Coronary artery bypass grafting
CAD	Coronary artery disease
CCU	Coronary care unit
CF	Colour flow
CFM	Colour flow mapping

CI	Cardiac index
CMR	Cardiac magnetic resonance imaging
CO	Cardiac output
CRT	Cardiac resynchronisation therapy
CRT-D	Cardiac resynchronisation therapy – defibrillator
CRT-P	Cardiac resynchronisation therapy – pacemaker
CSA	Cross-sectional area
CT	Computed tomography
CTRCD	Cancer therapy-related cardiac dysfunction
CVA	Cerebrovascular accident
CW	Continuous wave
DCM	Dilated cardiomyopathy
DT	Deceleration time
E_m (or e', E')	Early myocardial velocity
E:A	Ratio of E-wave to A-wave peak velocities
E-wave	Early wave of mitral flow
EACVI	European Association of Cardiovascular Imaging
EAE	European Association of Echocardiography
ECG	Electrocardiograph
Echo	Echocardiography/echocardiogram
EDTA	Ethylenediaminetetraacetic acid
EF	Ejection fraction
EMD	Electro-mechanical delay
EPS	Electrophysiological study
EROA	Effective regurgitant orifice area
ESC	European Society of Cardiology
ESR	Erythrocyte sedimentation rate
FS	Fractional shortening
FVI	Flow velocity integral
GA	General anaesthetic
HCM	Hypertrophic cardiomyopathy
HF	Heart failure
HIV	Human immunodeficiency virus
HOCM	Hypertrophic obstructive cardiomyopathy
IAS	Interatrial septum
ICD	Implantable cardioverter-defibrillator
ICS	Intercostal space
ICU	Intensive care unit
IE	Infective endocarditis
ITU	Intensive therapy unit
i.v.	Intravenous
IVC	Inferior vena cava
IVRT	Isovolumic relaxation time
IVS	Interventricular septum
IVSd	Interventricular septum thickness in diastole
IVSs	Interventricular septum thickness in systole
IVUS	Intravascular ultrasound

JVP	Jugular venous pressure
LA	Left atrium
LBBB	Left bundle branch block
LV	Left ventricle
LVEDD	Left ventricular end-diastolic diameter
LVEDP	Left ventricular end-diastolic pressure
LVEF	Left ventricular ejection fraction
LVESD	Left ventricular end-systolic diameter
LVH	Left ventricular hypertrophy
LVOT	Left ventricular outflow tract
LVOTO	Left ventricular outflow tract obstruction
LVPW	Left ventricular posterior wall
M-mode	Motion-mode
MAPSE	Mitral annular plane systolic excursion
MASV	Mitral annular systolic velocity
MI	Myocardial infarction
MR	Mitral regurgitation
MRI	Magnetic resonance imaging
MS	Mitral stenosis
MUGA	Multi-gated acquisition
MV	Mitral valve
MVA	Mitral valve area
MVP	Mitral valve prolapse
NICE	National Institute for Health and Care Excellence
NOAC	Novel oral anticoagulant
NT-proBNP	N-terminal pro-brain natriuretic peptide
NYHA	New York Heart Association
P_2	Pulmonary second sound
P-PEP	Pulmonary pre-ejection period
ΔP	Pressure gradient
PA	Pulmonary artery
PASP	Pulmonary artery systolic pressure
PCI	Percutaneous coronary intervention
PDA	Patent ductus arteriosus
PE	Pulmonary embolism
PFO	Patent foramen ovale
PHT	Pulmonary hypertension
PISA	Proximal isovelocity surface area
PLAX	Parasternal long-axis
PMVL	Posterior mitral valve leaflet
PR	Pulmonary regurgitation
PS	Pulmonary stenosis
PSAX	Parasternal short-axis
PV	Pulmonary valve
PW	Pulsed wave
RA	Right atrium
RAP	Right atrial pressure

RBBB	Right bundle branch block
RIHD	Radiation-induced heart disease
RPS	Right parasternal
RV	Right ventricle
RVEF	Right ventricular ejection fraction
RVOT	Right ventricular outflow tract
RVOTO	Right ventricular outflow tract obstruction
RVSP	Right ventricular systolic pressure
RWMA	Regional wall motion abnormality
S_1, S_2, etc.	First, second heart sounds, etc.
S_m (or s′, S′)	Systolic myocardial velocity
SAM	Systolic anterior motion
SBE	Subacute bacterial endocarditis
SC	Subcostal
SCD	Sudden cardiac death
SLE	Systemic lupus erythematosus
SPECT	Single-photon emission computed tomography
SSN	Suprasternal
STE	Speckle tracking echo
SV	Stroke volume
SVC	Superior vena cava
SVT	Supraventricular tachycardia
TAPSE	Tricuspid annular plane systolic excursion
TASV	Tricuspid annular systolic velocity
TAVI	Transcatheter aortic valve implantation
TAVR	Transcatheter aortic valve replacement
TDI	Tissue Doppler imaging
TIA	Transient ischaemic attack
TnI	Troponin I
TnT	Troponin T
TOE/TEE	Transoesophageal echocardiography
tPA	Tissue plasminogen activator
TR	Tricuspid regurgitation
TS	Tricuspid stenosis
TSI	Tissue synchronization imaging
TTE	Transthoracic echocardiography
TV	Tricuspid valve
V	Velocity
V_{max}	Maximum velocity
VEGF	Vascular endothelial growth factor
VF	Ventricular fibrillation
VSD	Ventricular septal defect
VT	Ventricular tachycardia
VTI	Velocity-time integral
WHO	World Health Organization

WHAT IS ECHO?

1.1 BASIC NOTIONS

Echocardiography (echo) – the use of ultrasound to examine the heart – is a safe, powerful, non-invasive and painless technique.

Echo is easy to understand as many features are based upon simple physical and physiological facts. It is a practical procedure requiring skill and is very operator dependent – the quality of the echo study and the information derived from it are influenced by who carries out the examination!

This chapter deals with:
• Ultrasound production and detection
• The echo techniques in common clinical use
• The normal echo
• Who should have an echo?

ULTRASOUND PRODUCTION AND DETECTION

Sound is a disturbance propagating in a material – air, water, body tissue or a solid substance. Each sound is characterized by its frequency and its intensity. Frequency is measured in hertz (Hz), that is, in oscillations per second, and its multiples (kilohertz, kHz, 10^3 Hz and megahertz, MHz, 10^6 Hz). Sound of frequency higher than 20 kHz cannot be perceived by the human ear and is called ultrasound. Echo uses ultrasound frequencies ranging from about 1.5 MHz to about 7.5 MHz. The nature of the material in which the sound propagates determines its velocity. In the heart, the velocity is 1540 m/s. The speed of sound in air is 330 m/s.

The wavelength of sound equals the ratio of velocity to frequency. In heart tissue, ultrasound with a frequency of 5 MHz has a wavelength of about 0.3 mm. The shorter the wavelength, the higher the resolution. As a rough estimate, the smallest size that can be resolved by a sound is equal to its wavelength. In contrast, the smaller the wavelength of the sound, the less its penetration power. Therefore, a compromise has to be made between resolution and penetration. A higher frequency of ultrasound can be used in children since less depth of penetration is needed.

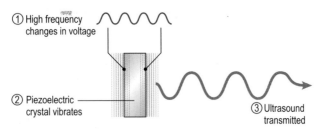

Figure 1.1 Piezoelectric effect.

Ultrasound results from the property of certain crystals to transform electrical oscillations (varying voltages) into mechanical oscillations (sound). This is called the piezoelectric effect (Fig. 1.1). The same crystals can also act as ultrasound receivers since they can effect the transformation in the opposite direction (mechanical to electrical).

The repetition rate is 1000/s. Each transmitting and receiving period lasts for 1 ms. Transmission accounts for 1 μs of this time. The remaining time is spent in 'receiving' mode.

At the core of any echo machine is this piezoelectric crystal transducer. When varying voltages are applied to the crystal, it vibrates and transmits ultrasound. When the crystal is in receiving mode, if it is struck by ultrasound waves, it is distorted. This generates an electrical signal that is analyzed by the echo machine. The crystal can receive as long as it is not transmitting at that time. This fixes the function of the crystal – it emits a pulse and then listens for a reflection.

When ultrasound propagates in a uniform medium, it maintains its initial direction and is progressively absorbed or scattered. If it meets a discontinuity, such as the interface of 2 parts of the medium having different densities, some of the ultrasound is reflected back. Ultrasound meets many tissue interfaces and echo reflections occur from different depths. Some interfaces or tissues are more echo-reflective than others (e.g. bone or calcium are more reflective than blood), and these appear as echo-bright reflections.

Two quantities are measured in an echo:
1. The time delay between transmission of the pulse and reception of the reflected echo
2. The intensity of the reflected signal, indicating the echo-reflectivity of that tissue or tissue–tissue interface.

The signals that return to the transducer give evidence of depth and intensity of reflection. These are transformed electronically into greyscale images on a monitor or printed on paper – high echo reflection is white, less reflection is grey and no reflection is black.

1.2 VIEWING THE HEART

Echo studies are carried out using specialized ultrasound machines. Ultrasound of different frequencies (in adults usually 2–4 MHz) is transmitted from a transducer (probe) that is placed on the subject's anterior chest wall. This is transthoracic echo (TTE). The transducer usually has a line or dot to help rotate it into the correct position to give different echo views. The subject usually lies in the left lateral position and ultrasound gel is placed on the transducer to ensure good images. Continuous electrocardiograph (ECG) recording is performed and phonocardiography may be used to time cardiac events. An echo examination usually takes 30–45 minutes (including reporting).

ECHO 'WINDOWS' AND VIEWS

There are several standard positions on the chest wall for the transducer where there are 'echo windows' that allow good penetration by ultrasound without too much masking and absorption by lung or ribs (Fig. 1.2).

A number of sections of the heart are examined by echo from these transducer positions, which are used for 2 main reasons:
1. There is a limitation determined by the anatomy of the heart and its surrounding structures
2. To produce standardized images that can be compared between different studies.

Useful echo information can be obtained in most subjects, but the study can be technically difficult in:
• Very obese subjects
• People with chest wall deformities

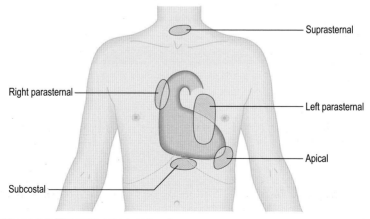

Figure 1.2 The main echo 'windows'.

- People with chronic lung disease (e.g. chronic airflow limitation with hyperinflated lungs or pulmonary fibrosis).

Rarely, an echo study is impossible.

A number of 'echo views' are obtained in most studies. 'Axis' refers to the plane in which the ultrasound beam travels through the heart.

Left parasternal window. (2nd-4th intercostal space, left sternal edge):

1. **Long-axis views** (Figs. 1.3, 1.4). Most examinations begin with a long-axis view. The transducer is used to obtain images of the heart in long axis, with slices from the base of the heart to the apex. The marker dot on the transducer points to the right shoulder. By angling the transducer, right ventricular (RV) inflow and outflow views can also be obtained.

2. **Short-axis views** (Figs. 1.5, 1.6). Without moving the transducer from its location on the chest wall and by rotating the transducer

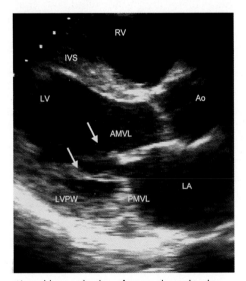

Figure 1.3 Parasternal long-axis view. Arrows show chordae.

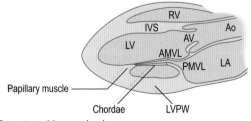

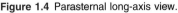

Figure 1.4 Parasternal long-axis view.

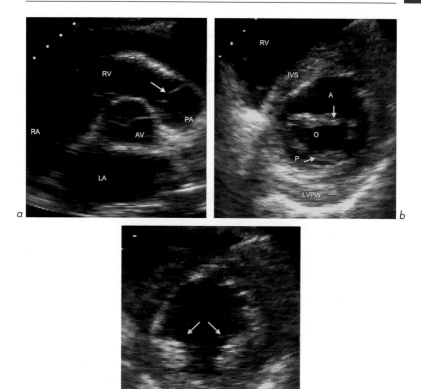

Figure 1.5 Parasternal short-axis views: **(a)** Aortic valve level. The pulmonary valve is shown (arrow). **(b)** Mitral valve level. The anterior (A) and posterior (P) leaflets are shown. Mitral orifice (O). **(c)** Papillary muscles (arrows) level.

through 90° so the marker dot is pointing towards the left shoulder, the heart is cut in transverse (short-axis) sections. By changing the angulation on the chest wall, it is possible to obtain any number of short-axis views, but the standard 4 are at the level of the aortic valve (AV), mitral valve (MV), left ventricular papillary muscles and left ventricular apex (Figs. 1.5, 1.6).

Apical window. (Cardiac apex):

1. **4-chamber view** (Figs. 1.7a, 1.8a). The transducer is placed at the cardiac apex with the marker dot pointing down towards the left shoulder. This gives the typical 'heart-shaped' 4-chamber view (Fig. 1.7a).

2. **5-chamber (including aortic outflow)** (Figs. 1.7b, 1.8b). By altering the angulation of the transducer so the ultrasound beam is angled

Parasternal short-axis views

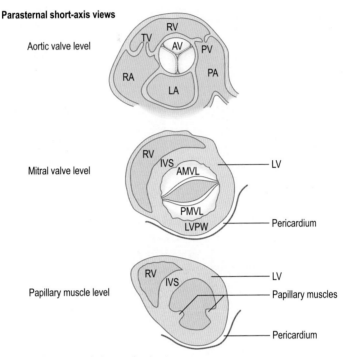

Figure 1.6 Parasternal short-axis views.

more anteriorly towards the chest wall, a '5-chamber' view is obtained. The 5th 'chamber' is not a chamber at all but is the AV and ascending aorta. This is useful in assessing aortic stenosis (AS) and aortic regurgitation (AR).

3. **Long-axis (3-chamber) and 2-chamber views** (Figs. 1.7c, 1.8c, 1.8d). By rotating the transducer on the cardiac apex, it is possible to obtain apical long-axis and 2-chamber views, which show different segments of the left ventricle (LV).

Subcostal window. (Under the xiphisternum) (Figs. 1.9, 1.10):
Similar views to apical views, but rotated by approximately 90°. Useful in lung disease, in people with poor parasternal and apical windows, for imaging the interatrial septum, and for assessing pericardial fluid collection (effusion), the inferior vena cava (IVC) and the abdominal aorta.

Further windows may be used:

Suprasternal window. (Imaging from above the suprasternal notch) (Fig. 1.11):
For imaging the ascending aorta, arch and descending aorta (e.g. in aortic coarctation).

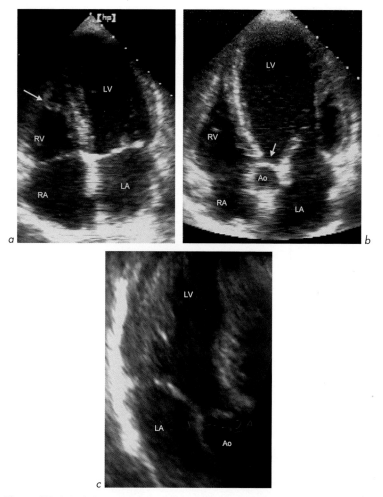

Figure 1.7 Apical views: **(a)** Apical 4-chamber view. A moderator band is shown (arrow). This is a normal neuromuscular bundle carrying right bundle branch fibres. **(b)** Apical 5-chamber view. The aortic valve is shown (arrow). **(c)** Apical long-axis view.

Right parasternal window. (2nd-3rd intercostal space, right sternal edge):
 In aortic stenosis (AS) and to examine the ascending aorta.

1.3 ECHO TECHNIQUES

Three echo methods are in common clinical usage (see Table 1.1 for typical applications):
• Two-dimensional (2-D) or 'cross-sectional'
• Motion or M-mode

a 4-chamber

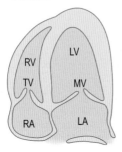

c 2-chamber

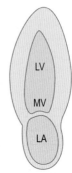

b 5-chamber

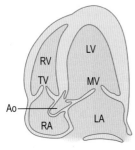

d Long-axis

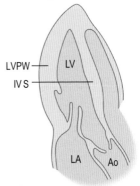

Figure 1.8 Apical views.

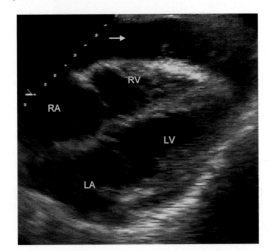

Figure 1.9 Subcostal 4-chamber view. A pericardial effusion is seen (arrow).

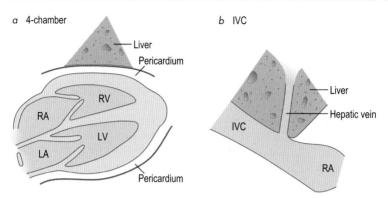

Figure 1.10 Subcostal views. **(a)** 4-chamber view. **(b)** Inferior vena cava (IVC) view.

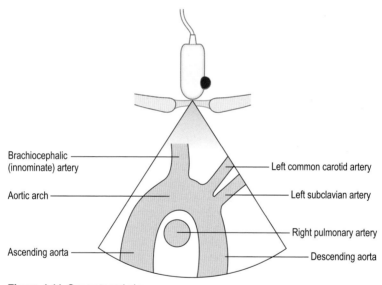

Figure 1.11 Suprasternal view.

- Doppler – continuous wave (CW), pulsed wave (PW) and colour flow.

2-D echo gives a snapshot in time of a cross-section of tissue. If these sections are produced in quick succession and displayed on a monitor, they can show 'real-time imaging' of the heart chambers, valves and blood vessels.

To create a 2-D image, the ultrasound beam must be swept across the area of interest. The transducer rotates the beam it produces through a certain angle, either mechanically or electronically (Fig. 1.12). In the first case, the transducer is rotated so that its beam scans

Table 1.1 Summary of echo modalities and their main uses

2-D echo	• Anatomy • Ventricular and valvular movement • Positioning for M-mode and Doppler echo
M-mode echo	• Measurement of dimensions • Timing cardiac events
Pulsed wave Doppler	• Normal valve flow patterns • LV diastolic function • Stroke volume and cardiac output
Continuous wave Doppler	• Severity of valvular stenosis • Severity of valvular regurgitation • Velocity of flow in shunts
Colour flow mapping	• Assessment of regurgitation and shunts

the target. In the second case, several crystals are mounted together and are excited by voltages in sequence. Each crystal emits waves. The result is a summation wave that moves in a direction determined by the 'phased stimulation' of the crystals. The reflected ultrasound generates an electrical signal in the crystal, which is used to produce a dot on the monitor. Ultrasound is transmitted along scan lines (usually about 120 lines) over an arc of approximately 90° at least 20–30 times per second and in some newer systems up to 120 times per second. Reflected ultrasound signals are combined on the monitor to build up a moving image. Frozen images can be printed out on paper or photographic film.

Motion or M-mode echo (Fig. 1.13) is produced by the transmission and reception of an ultrasound signal along only one line, giving high sensitivity (greater than 2-D echo) for recording moving structures. It produces a graph of depth and strength of reflection with time. Changes in movement (e.g. valve opening and closing or ventricular wall movement) can be displayed. The ultrasound signal should be aligned perpendicularly to the structure being examined. Measurement of the size and thickness of cardiac chambers can be made either manually on paper printouts or on the monitor using computer software.

Doppler echo uses the reflection of ultrasound by moving red blood cells. The Doppler principle is used to derive velocity information (Chapter 3). The reflected ultrasound has a frequency shift relative to the transmitted ultrasound, determined by the velocity and direction of blood flow. This gives haemodynamic information regarding the heart and blood vessels. It can be used to measure the severity of valvular narrowing (stenosis), to detect valvular leakage (regurgitation) and can show intracardiac shunts such as ventricular septal defects (VSDs) and atrial septal defects (ASDs) (Chapter 6).

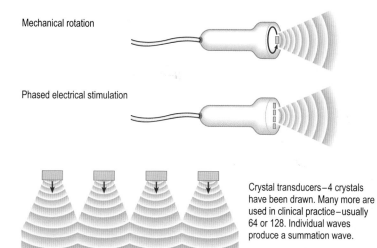

Mechanical rotation

Phased electrical stimulation

Crystal transducers – 4 crystals have been drawn. Many more are used in clinical practice – usually 64 or 128. Individual waves produce a summation wave.

Figure 1.12 Mechanical and electronic transducers.

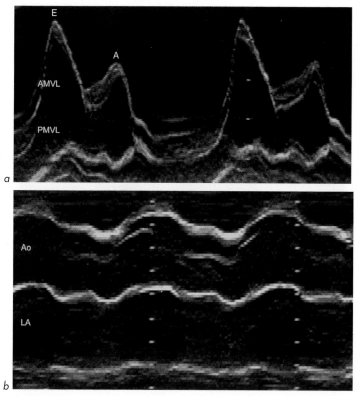

Figure 1.13 M-mode patterns. **(a)** Mitral valve and **(b)** Aortic root and left atrium.

The 3 commonly used Doppler echo techniques are:

1. **Continuous wave (CW) Doppler.** Two crystals are used – one transmitting continuously and one receiving continuously. This technique is useful for measuring high velocities but its ability to localize a flow signal precisely is limited since the signal can originate at any point along the length or width of the ultrasound beam (Fig. 1.14).

2. **Pulsed wave (PW) Doppler** (Fig. 1.15). This allows a flow disturbance to be localized or blood velocity from a small region to be measured. A single crystal is used to transmit an ultrasound signal and then to receive after a pre-set time delay. Reflected signals are only recorded from a depth corresponding to half the product of the time delay and the speed of sound in tissues (1540 m/s). By combining this technique with 2-D imaging, a small 'sample volume' can be identified on the screen showing the region where velocities are being measured. The operator can move the sample volume. Because the time delay limits the rate at which sampling can occur, there is a limit to the maximum velocity that can be accurately detected, before a phenomenon known as 'aliasing' occurs, usually at velocities in excess of 2 m/s. The theoretical limit of the sampling rate is known as the Nyquist frequency (or limit). This is equal to half of the pulse repetition frequency.

CW and PW Doppler allow a graphical representation of velocity against time and are also referred to as 'spectral Doppler'.

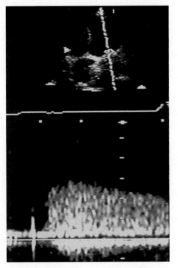

Figure 1.14 Continuous wave Doppler of severe mitral stenosis. Mean gradient 20 mmHg.

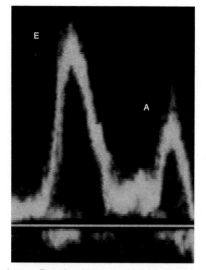

Figure 1.15 Pulsed wave Doppler. Normal mitral flow pattern.

3. **Colour flow mapping (CFM).** This is an automated 2-D version of PW Doppler. It calculates blood velocity and direction at multiple points along a number of scan lines superimposed on a 2-D echo image. The velocities and directions of blood flow are colour-encoded. Velocities away from the transducer are in blue, those towards it in red. This is known as the BART convention (Blue Away, Red Towards). Higher velocities are shown in progressively lighter shades of colour. Above a threshold velocity, 'colour reversal' occurs (explained again by the phenomenon of aliasing). Areas of high turbulence or regions of high flow acceleration are often indicated in green (Fig. 1.16).

A detailed description of echo views and techniques is given in Chapter 8, 'Performing and reporting an echo'.

1.4 THE NORMAL ECHO

Echo provides a great deal of anatomical and haemodynamic information:
• Heart chamber size
• Chamber function (systolic and diastolic)
• Valvular motion and function
• Intracardiac and extracardiac masses and fluid collections
• Direction of blood flow and haemodynamic information (e.g. valvular stenosis and pressure gradients) by Doppler echo.

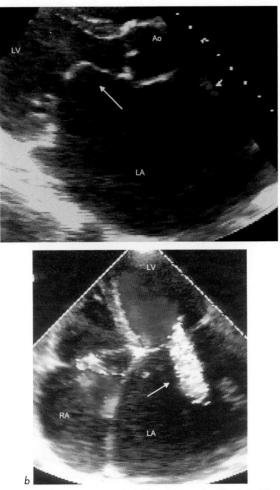

Figure 1.16 Rheumatic mitral regurgitation and stenosis. The left atrium is very enlarged. **(a)** The anterior leaflet shows 'elbowing' (arrow) on parasternal long-axis view. **(b)** A jet of mitral regurgitation is seen (arrow) on colour flow mapping in the apical 4-chamber view.

'NORMAL ECHO RANGES'

It is important to remember that these 'normal ranges' vary with a number of factors. The frequently quoted values of, e.g. left atrial diameter or left ventricular cavity internal dimensions, do not take this into account. Important factors which influence cardiac dimensions measured by echo are:
- Height
- Sex

- Age
- Physical training (athletes)
- Ethnicity
- Obesity.

In general, values are higher in taller individuals, males and athletes. Some correction for these factors can be made, for example, in very tall individuals, by indexing the measurement to body surface area (BSA):

$$BSA\ (m^2) = \sqrt{\frac{height\ (cm) \times weight\ (kg)}{3600}}$$

Bearing these points in mind, it is useful to have an indication of some *approximate* echo-derived 'normal values' (Table 1.2).

Some other findings on echo may be normal:

1. Mild tricuspid regurgitation (TR) and mitral regurgitation (MR) are found in many normal hearts.
2. Some degree of thickening of AV leaflets with ageing is normal without significant AS. This is called aortic sclerosis.
3. Mitral annulus (ring) calcification is sometimes seen in older people. It is often of no consequence but may be misdiagnosed as a stenosed valve, a vegetation (inflammatory mass), thrombus (clot) or myxoma (cardiac tumour). It is important to examine the leaflets carefully. It may be associated with MR (Fig. 1.17).
4. An 'upper septal bulge' (Fig. 1.18) is common, particularly in older women, and should not be misdiagnosed as hypertrophic cardiomyopathy (HCM). It is due to septal hypertrophy and fibrosis and only rarely causes significant LV outflow tract obstruction (LVOTO).
5. In the atria, there may be:
   - Chiari network. Found in 1.3–4% of individuals. An embryological remnant of the right valve of the sinus venosus. On echo, this can be seen as a highly mobile, web-like, filamentous, wafting and very reflective structure in the right atrium (RA). It is attached to the RA wall close to the junction with the IVC. It can be mistaken for a vegetation, thrombus or tumour.
   - Eustachian valve. An endocardial ridge or fold, at the junction of the IVC and RA. In the fetal heart, it directs blood towards the foramen ovalis. It has no function in adults. It can be mistaken on echo for tumour, thrombus or vegetation
   - Crista terminalis. This is a muscular ridge, which passes anteriorly from superior vena cava (SVC) to IVC. It is a remnant that marks the site of fusion of the embryological RA (which later becomes the RA appendage) with the sinus venosus

Table 1.2 'Normal values' for adults – based on American Society of Echocardiography (ASE) guidelines 2015

			Women	Men
Left ventricle (LV)				
Internal diameter	End-diastolic diameter (LVEDD)	–	3.8–5.2 cm	4.2–5.8 cm
	End-systolic diameter (LVESD)	–	2.2–3.5 cm	2.5–4.0 cm
Wall thickness	End-diastolic	Interventricular septum	0.6–0.9 cm	0.6–1.0 cm
		Posterior wall	0.6–0.9 cm	0.6–1.0 cm
	End-systolic	Interventricular septum	0.9–1.8 cm	0.9–1.8 cm
		Posterior wall	0.9–1.8 cm	0.9–1.8 cm
Ejection fraction	–	–	54–74%	52–72%
Fractional shortening	–	–	27–45%	25–43%
Left atrium (LA)				
Diameter	–	–	2.7–3.8 cm	3.0–4.0 cm
Aortic root*				
Sinuses of Valsalva diameter	–	–	2.7–3.3 cm	3.1–3.7 cm
Ascending aorta diameter	–	–	2.3–3.1 cm	2.6–3.4 cm
Right ventricle (RV)				
Internal diameter	Basal RV	End-diastolic	2.5–4.1 cm	2.5–4.1 cm
	Mid-RV	End-diastolic	1.9–3.5 cm	1.9–3.5 cm
RV outflow tract diameter	Proximal (RV to AV)	End-diastolic (parasternal short-axis view)	2.1–3.5 cm	2.1–3.5 cm
	Distal (proximal to PV)	End-diastolic (parasternal short-axis view)	1.7–2.7 cm	1.7–2.7 cm
Wall thickness	End-diastolic	–	0.1–0.5 cm	0.1–0.5 cm

Most values are derived from M-mode measurements in parasternal long-axis view.
*See also Section 6.5. Based upon Lang et al. J Am Soc Echocardiogr. 2015;28:1–39.

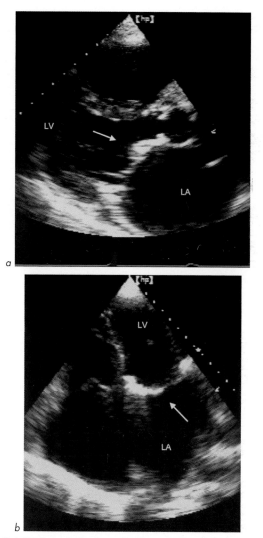

Figure 1.17 Calcification of mitral annulus (arrow). This was asymptomatic, with no mitral stenosis or regurgitation. **(a)** Parasternal long-axis view. **(b)** Apical 4-chamber view.

derived portion of the RA. It can be mistaken on echo for tumour, thrombus or vegetation.

- Lipomatous hypertrophy of interatrial septum. Thickening due to deposits of fatty material, which may be localized or generalized (fossa ovalis is spared). When localized, it may be mistaken on echo for tumour, thrombus or vegetation.

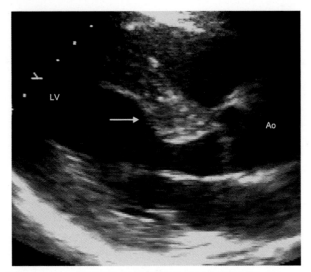

Figure 1.18 Upper septal bulge (arrow). Parasternal long-axis view.

1.5 WHO SHOULD HAVE AN ECHO?

In order to obtain the most useful information, it is essential to provide:
• Adequate clinical information
• The reason an echo is being requested
• The specific question being asked.

Examples: '60-year-old man with breathlessness and previous anterior myocardial infarction, awaiting general anaesthesia for elective hip replacement surgery – please assess LV systolic function', or, '70-year-old woman with aortic ejection systolic murmur – please assess severity of aortic stenosis.'

The following list of indications is not exhaustive and others are found in the relevant sections of the book. The list gives situations in which an echo may influence the clinical management of a patient:
• Assessment of valve function, e.g. systolic or diastolic murmur
• Assessment of left ventricular function – systolic, diastolic and regional wall motion, e.g. suspected heart failure in a person with breathlessness or oedema, or preoperative assessment
• Suspected endocarditis
• Suspected myocarditis
• Cardiac tamponade
• Pericardial disease (e.g. pericarditis) or pericardial effusion, especially if clinical evidence of tamponade

- Complications of myocardial infarction (MI), e.g. VSD, MR, effusion
- Suspicion of intracardiac masses – tumour, thrombus
- Cardiac chamber size, e.g. left atrium (LA) in atrial fibrillation (AF), cardiomegaly on chest X-ray
- Assessment of artificial (prosthetic) valve function
- Arrhythmias, e.g. AF, ventricular tachycardia (VT)
- Assessment of RV and right heart
- Estimation of intracardiac and vascular pressures, e.g. pulmonary artery systolic pressure (PASP) in lung disease and suspected pulmonary hypertension (PHT)
- Stroke and transient ischaemic attack (TIA) – 'cardiac source of embolism?'
- Exclusion of left ventricular hypertrophy (LVH) in hypertension
- Assessment of congenital heart disease.

1.6 MURMURS

A murmur is a sound caused by turbulent blood flow. It may be caused by:
- High velocity or volume across a normal valve
- Forward flow across a diseased valve
- Leakage across a valve
- Flow through a shunt (an abnormal communication between chambers or vessels)
- Flow across a narrowed blood vessel.

Echo helps to diagnose the underlying cause of a murmur and the severity of the haemodynamic effect, and to plan treatment.

1. POSSIBLE CAUSES OF A SYSTOLIC MURMUR

- Benign flow murmur – features suggesting this are short, ejection, mid-systolic, soft or moderate in loudness, normal second heart sound, may be louder on inspiration or on lying flat
- Aortic – 'sclerosis' or stenosis
- HCM
- Mitral – regurgitation, prolapse
- Pulmonary – stenosis
- Tricuspid – regurgitation (rarely heard – diagnosis made by seeing systolic waves in jugular venous pressure [JVP])
- Shunts – intracardiac or extracardiac – congenital, e.g. ASD (high flow across pulmonary valve [PV]), VSD, patent ductus arteriosus (PDA) or acquired (e.g. post-MI VSD)
- Coarctation of the aorta.

2. CONDITIONS ASSOCIATED WITH A BENIGN SYSTOLIC MURMUR

(NO underlying cardiac disease) – common in childhood and pregnancy.
- Pulmonary flow – common, especially in young children (30%)
- Venous hum – continuous, reduced by neck vein compression, turning head laterally, bending elbows or lying down. Loudest in neck and around clavicles
- Mammary souffle – particularly in pregnancy
- High-flow states – pregnancy, anaemia, fever, anxiety, thyrotoxicosis (although in the case of thyrotoxicosis there may be associated cardiac disease).

3. POSSIBLE CAUSES OF A DIASTOLIC MURMUR

Abnormal – except venous hum or mammary souffle:
- Aortic – regurgitation
- Mitral – stenosis
- Pulmonary – regurgitation
- Tricuspid – stenosis (rare)
- Congenital shunts – e.g. PDA.

4. WHO WITH A MURMUR SHOULD HAVE AN ECHO?

Features suggesting a murmur is pathological/organic

An echo should be requested for anyone whose murmur is not clearly clinically benign (e.g. pulmonary flow, venous hum, mammary souffle), especially if there are any features of a pathological murmur:
- Symptoms – chest pain, breathlessness, oedema, syncope, dizziness, palpitations
- Cyanosis
- Thrill (palpable murmur)
- Diastolic murmur*
- Pansystolic*
- Very loud murmur (but remember – the *loudness* of a murmur often bears no relation to the *severity* of the valve lesion)
- Added/abnormal heart sounds – abnormal S_2, ejection clicks, opening snaps, S_4 (not S_3, which can be normal, particularly if age <30 years)
- Physical signs of heart failure
- Wide pulse pressure and displaced apex
- Suspected endocarditis
- Suspected aortic dissection
- Cardiomegaly (e.g. on chest X-ray)
- Associated ECG abnormalities, e.g. LVH.

(*Exceptions are venous hum or mammary souffle as above.)

VALVES

2.1 MITRAL VALVE (MV)

One of the earliest applications of echo was in the diagnosis of valvular heart disease, particularly mitral stenosis (MS). M-mode echo still provides very useful information, nowadays complemented by 2-D and Doppler techniques.

The MV is located between the LA and LV. The MV opens during ventricular diastole when blood flows from LA into LV. During ventricular systole, the MV closes as blood is ejected through AV.

The MV has 3 main components:
- Leaflets (2) – anterior and posterior
- Chordae attached to papillary muscles ('subvalvular apparatus')
- Annulus (valve ring).

The 2 leaflets are attached at one end to the annulus and at the other (free) edge to the chordae, which are fixed to the LV by the papillary muscles. The chordae hold each of the MV leaflets like cords hold a parachute canopy. The leaflets' free edges meet at 2 points called the commissures (Figs. 2.1, 2.2).

Movement of the MV leaflets can be seen by M-mode and 2-D echo. The normal MV leaflets have a characteristic movement pattern on M-mode examination. The anterior MV leaflet (AMVL) sweeps an M-shape pattern, whilst the posterior MV leaflet (PMVL) sweeps a W-shaped pattern (Fig. 1.13a). Understanding the origin of the normal MV opening and closing pattern is easy and helps in understanding abnormal patterns in disease (Fig. 2.3).

The first peak of MV movement (early, E-wave) coincides with passive LA to LV flow. The second peak coincides with atrial contraction and active flow of blood into the LV (atrial, A-wave). This pattern of movement is brought about by the characteristics of blood flow into the LV. This second peak is lost in AF, where atrial mechanical activity is absent. On 2-D examination, the normal MV leaflets should be thin, mobile and separate and close well. Their motion should be of a double waveform as expected from the M-mode findings. The Doppler pattern of mitral flow shows a similar pattern to M-mode movement of the MV leaflets.

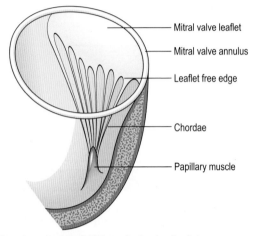

Mitral valve leaflet
Mitral valve annulus
Leaflet free edge
Chordae
Papillary muscle

Figure 2.1 Attachment of one of the mitral valve leaflets.

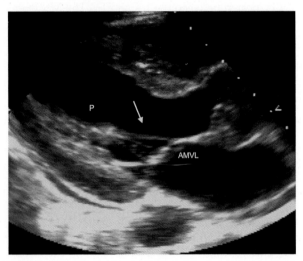

Figure 2.2 Part of the mitral valve apparatus. Anterior mitral valve leaflet (AMVL), papillary muscle (P) and chordae tendineae (arrow).

MITRAL STENOSIS (MS)

In practical terms, the only common cause of MS is **rheumatic heart disease.**

Much rarer causes include mitral annulus calcification (usually asymptomatic and more likely to be associated with MR, rarely stenosis), congenital (may be associated with congenital AS or aortic coarctation), connective tissue disorders and infiltrations, systemic lupus erythematosus (SLE), rheumatoid arthritis, mucopolysaccharidoses (Hurler's syndrome) and carcinoid.

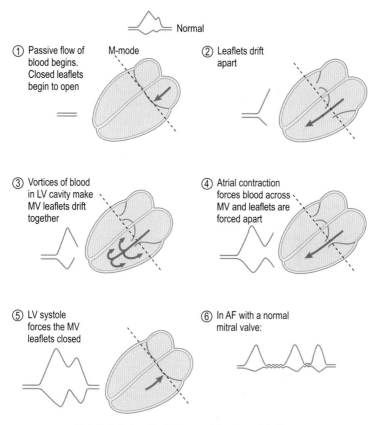

① Passive flow of
blood begins.
Closed leaflets
begin to open

M-mode

Normal

② Leaflets drift
apart

③ Vortices of blood
in LV cavity make
MV leaflets drift
together

④ Atrial contraction
forces blood across
MV and leaflets are
forced apart

⑤ LV systole
forces the MV
leaflets closed

⑥ In AF with a normal
mitral valve:

Note that similar effects happen at the tricuspid valve

Figure 2.3 Origin of the M-mode pattern of normal mitral valve opening and closing.

Rheumatic fever is an autoimmune phenomenon caused by cross-reaction of antibodies to streptococcal bacterial antigens with antigens found on the heart. In its acute stages, rheumatic fever is associated with inflammation of all layers of the heart – endocardium (including those of the valves), myocardium and pericardium. MS does not occur at this stage, but many years later as a consequence of this initial inflammatory process. The MV leaflets progressively fuse, initially at the commissures and free edges, which become thickened and later calcified. The inflamed valve becomes progressively thickened, fibrosed and calcified. This restricts the opening and closing of the valve. The chordae may also become thickened, shortened and calcified, further restricting normal valve function. The leaflets shrink and become rigid. The size of the MV orifice reduces leading to MS, which restricts blood flow from the LA to the LV.

Remember that many years elapse between rheumatic fever and the clinical manifestations of MS but there may not be a clear clinical history of rheumatic fever in childhood. Some individuals may remember being placed on bedrest for many weeks, which was the often-favoured treatment for rheumatic fever.

The **M-mode** pattern changes in a predictable way (Fig. 2.4). The movement of the leaflets is more restricted, and the leaflet tips are fused, so the posterior leaflet is pulled towards the anterior leaflet rather than drifting away from it. In severe MS, there is often AF rather than sinus rhythm, and the second peak of MV movement is lost. The calcified leaflets reflect ultrasound in a different pattern from normal leaflets due to their increased thickness, fibrosis and often calcification. Instead of a single echo reflection giving a sharp image of the leaflets, there is a reverberation with several echo reflections giving a fuzzy image. Calcified leaflets produce a stronger echo reflection.

On **2-D echo**, the MV leaflets are thickened and their movement restricted. Because of the fusion of the anterior and posterior leaflet

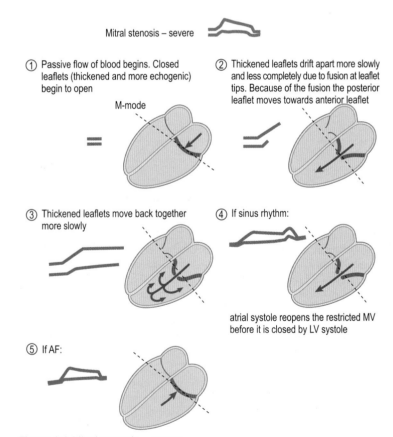

Mitral stenosis – severe

① Passive flow of blood begins. Closed leaflets (thickened and more echogenic) begin to open

M-mode

② Thickened leaflets drift apart more slowly and less completely due to fusion at leaflet tips. Because of the fusion the posterior leaflet moves towards anterior leaflet

③ Thickened leaflets move back together more slowly

④ If sinus rhythm:

atrial systole reopens the restricted MV before it is closed by LV systole

⑤ If AF:

Figure 2.4 Mitral stenosis – severe.

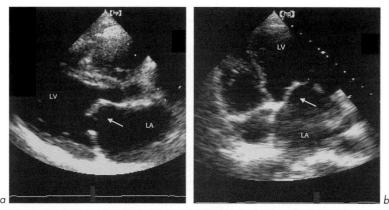

Figure 2.5 Rheumatic mitral stenosis. **(a)** Parasternal long-axis view and **(b)** apical 4-chamber view. 'Elbowing' of the anterior mitral valve leaflet is shown (arrow).

tips, whilst the leaflet cusps may remain relatively mobile, there may be a characteristic 'elbowing' or 'bent-knee' appearance, particularly of the anterior MV leaflet (Figs. 2.5, 2.6). This has also been likened to the bulging of a boat's sail as it fills with wind. The LA also enlarges.

The computer of the echo machine can calculate the area of the MV orifice after tracing around a frozen image on a parasternal short-axis view taken at the level of the MV leaflets in end-diastole. The normal leaflets in this view open and close in a 'fish-mouth' pattern. In MS, the leaflet tips are calcified and opening is restricted with a reduced orifice size.

MV orifice area (Fig. 2.7) can also be measured using Doppler (Chapter 3).

Changes in MV area with severity of MS

- Normal valve　4.0–6.0 cm^2
- Mild MS　　　1.6–3.9 cm^2
- Moderate MS　1.0–1.5 cm^2
- Severe MS　　< 1.0 cm^2.

Criteria for diagnosis of severe MS (many derived from Doppler)

- Measured valve orifice area <1.0 cm^2
- Mean pressure gradient >10 mmHg
- Pressure half-time >200 ms
- Pulmonary artery systolic pressure (PASP) >50 mmHg.

For severity of MS see Table 2.1.

Parasternal long-axis view

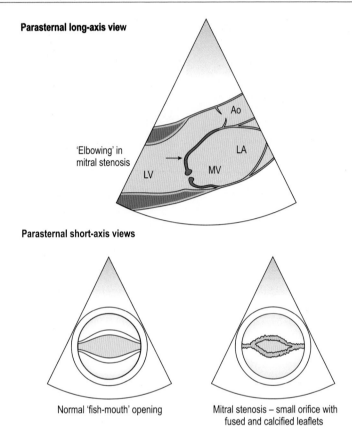

Parasternal short-axis views

Normal 'fish-mouth' opening

Mitral stenosis – small orifice with fused and calcified leaflets

Figure 2.6 2-D echo in mitral stenosis.

A number of diseases produce other typical mitral **M-mode** patterns (Fig. 2.8):

- *LA myxoma.* This has a characteristic appearance. There are multiple echoes filling the space between the MV leaflets. There may initially be an echo-free zone that is filled with echo reflections as the myxoma prolapses through the MV from LA into LV. Other potential causes of a similar echo appearance are large MV vegetations, LA thrombus or aneurysm of the MV.
- *Hypertrophic cardiomyopathy (HCM).* In diastole, the valve may be normal, but in systole the entire MV apparatus moves anteriorly producing a characteristic bulge touching the IVS. This is called systolic anterior motion (SAM) of the MV.
- *MV prolapse.* This may be asymptomatic or cause varying degrees of MR. Either anterior or posterior valve leaflets may prolapse into the LA cavity in late systole. This produces an audible click and a late systolic murmur.

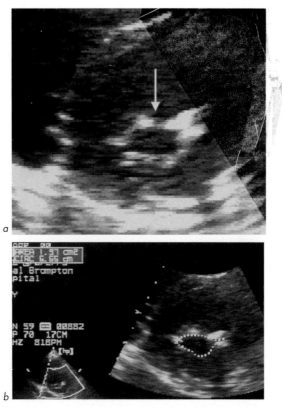

Figure 2.7 Rheumatic mitral stenosis. **(a)** Parasternal short-axis view at mitral level showing restricted orifice (arrow) and **(b)** valve orifice area calculated by computer software as 1.9 cm².

Table 2.1 Assessment of severity of mitral stenosis (MS) – based upon EAE/ASE guidelines

	Mild	Moderate	Severe
Valve area	>1.5 cm²	1.0–1.5 cm²	<1.0 cm²
Mean gradient	<5 mmHg	5–10 mmHg	>10 mmHg
PA pressure	<30 mmHg	30–50 mmHg	>50 mmHg

Based on data from Baumgartner H, Hung J, Bermejo J, et al. Echocardiographic assessment of valve stenosis: EAE/ASE recommendations for clinical practice. Eur J Echocardiogr. 2009;10:1–25.

- *Flail posterior leaflet.* This may occur as a result of chordal rupture (due to degeneration) or to papillary muscle dysfunction. The posterior leaflet shows erratic movement, rather than the normal 'W' pattern.
- *Aortic regurgitation (AR).* The regurgitant jet passes during diastole along the anterior MV leaflet, causing fluttering vibration of the

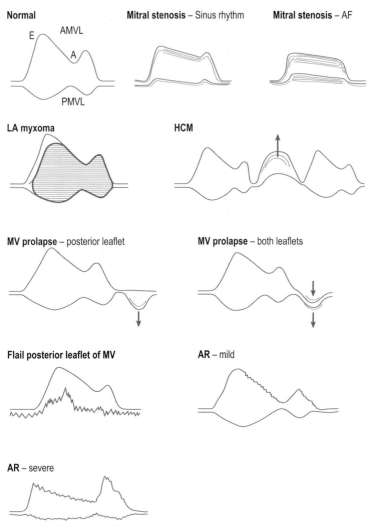

Figure 2.8 Mitral valve M-mode patterns.

leaflet and restricting its normal pattern of movement. With increasing severity of AR, the MV is more restricted and there may be 'functional' MS (with an anatomically normal MV) giving rise to the diastolic Austin Flint murmur.

MITRAL REGURGITATION (MR)

This is leakage of blood through the MV from the LV into the LA during ventricular systole. It ranges from very mild to very severe, when the majority of the LV volume empties into the LA rather than into the aorta with each cardiac cycle. A small amount of MR occurs during the closure of many normal MVs – in some series in up to one-third of normal hearts.

In MR, there are changes in:
- The function of the MV
- The LV, which becomes dilated, volume-overloaded and hyperdynamic to maintain cardiac output, since a large proportion of each stroke volume is regurgitating into the LA
- The LA, which becomes dilated.

Echo may show:
- An underlying MV abnormality, for example, flail MV leaflet with chaotic movement, MV prolapse, vegetations
- Rapid diastolic MV closure due to rapid filling
- Dilated LV with rapid filling (dimensions relate to prognosis)
- Septal and posterior wall motion becomes more vigorous
- Increased circumferential fibre shortening with good LV function
- LA size increased
- Doppler shows size and site of regurgitant jet.

Echo assessment of severity of MR

Whilst the diagnosis of MR may be easy (Fig. 2.9), the echo assessment of severity can be difficult. A balance must be made of all the echo information. The severity relates to the regurgitant fraction, which depends on:
- The size of the regurgitant orifice
- The length of time for which it remains open
- The systolic pressure difference between the LV and the LA across the valve
- The distensibility of the LA.

The features of severe chronic MR are those of:
1. Volume overload of the LV – dilatation with hyperdynamic movement
2. Volume overload of the LA – dilatation
3. Large regurgitant volume – broad jet extending far into the LA
4. Abnormal valve function.

M-mode shows LV dimensions are increased, as is velocity of motion of the posterior wall and interventricular septum (IVS). The LA is enlarged. There may be features of an underlying cause of MR, for example, multiple echoes suggesting vegetations due to endocarditis, MV prolapse or flail posterior leaflet.

2-D echo helps to suggest an underlying cause and assess its consequences. The parasternal long- and short-axis views and apical 4-chamber views are the most helpful and may show:
1. LV abnormality – dilatation causing annular stretching and 'functional' MR, regional wall motion abnormality due to MI or ischaemia, volume-overloaded LV

Chronic MR

1. Leaflet abnormalities
- rheumatic heart disease – usually in association with mitral stenosis
- MV prolapse ('floppy mitral valve')
- endocarditis
- connective tissue disorders – Marfan's, Ehlers–Danlos, pseudoxanthoma elasticum, osteogenesis imperfecta, SLE
- trauma
- congenital – cleft MV or parachute MV

2. Annulus abnormalities
(circumference usually 10 cm)
- dilatation due to LV dysfunction, e.g. dilated cardiomyopathy or following myocardial infarction. This causes 'functional' MR
- annular calcification – idiopathic, increasing with age, or associated with other conditions, e.g. hypertension, diabetes, aortic stenosis, hypertrophic cardiomyopathy (HCM), hyperparathyroidism, Marfan's

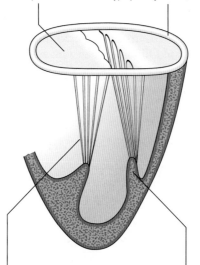

3. Abnormalities of the chordae tendineae
(rupture – more commonly the posterior leaflet)
- idiopathic
- endocarditis
- rheumatic heart disease
- mitral valve prolapse
- Marfan's
- osteogenesis imperfecta

4. Papillary muscle abnormalities
- ischaemia or infarction
- LV dilatation
- rheumatic heart disease
- HCM
- infiltration – sarcoid, amyloid
- myocarditis

Acute MR
- acute myocardial infarction (papillary muscle dysfunction or infarction)
- endocarditis
- chordal rupture

Figure 2.9 Causes of mitral regurgitation.

2. Leaflet abnormalities – rheumatic leaflets, vegetations due to endocarditis, prolapse, flail leaflet

3. Chordae – rupture, thickening, shortening, calcification, vegetations

4. Papillary muscles – rupture, hypertrophy, scarring, calcification.

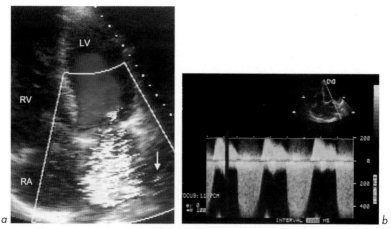

Figure 2.10 Severe mitral regurgitation. **(a)** Colour flow mapping shows a broad jet filling the left atrium and extending into pulmonary veins (arrow). **(b)** Continuous wave Doppler.

Doppler echo features of severe MR (Figs. 2.10, 5.6):

1. Wide jet. The width of the MR jet at the level of the leaflet tips (broad colour flow signal) correlates with severity (a wider jet represents more severe MR). This is called the vena contracta (the narrowest diameter of the jet flow stream that occurs at or just downstream from the orifice).

2. Jet fills a large area of LA. The extent to which the MR jet fills the LA cavity is also an indication. The area of colour in the LA depends on the machine settings and is controversial. However, an area >10 cm^2 is likely to be severe and <4 cm^2 is likely to be mild.

3. Systolic flow reversal in pulmonary veins. The jet extends to the pulmonary veins. This can be seen on colour flow mapping and may also cause retrograde flow (LA to the lungs) detected by pulsed wave Doppler with the sample volume in one of the pulmonary veins.

4. Dense signal on continuous Doppler. The intensity of the jet is greater with more severe MR since more red cells reflect ultrasound.

5. Raised PA pressure. This is estimated by Doppler from tricuspid regurgitation (TR) (Chapter 3).

It is important to know that severe *acute* MR (e.g. due to papillary muscle rupture in acute MI) may not have all of these echo features. There is not the time for the features of LV and LA dilatation to develop. A recently occurring narrow high velocity jet of MR into a normal-sized LA may cause a significant rise in LA pressure and symptoms such as breathlessness and signs such as acute pulmonary oedema.

American Society of Echocardiography (ASE) guidelines to assess severity of MR are shown in Table 2.2.

Table 2.2 Severity of mitral regurgitation (MR) – based upon ASE guidelines

	Mild	Moderate	Severe
Vena contracta diameter*	<0.3 cm	0.3–0.7 cm	>0.7 cm
Regurgitant volume	<30 mL	30–59 mL	>60 mL
Regurgitant fraction	<30%	30–49%	>50%
Regurgitant orifice area	<0.2 cm^2	0.2–0.39 cm^2	>0.4 cm^2
PISA lite radius**	<0.4 cm	0.4–1.0 cm	>1.0 cm
Colour flow jet area	<4 cm^2 or <20% LA area	4–10 cm^2 or 20–40% LA area	>10 cm^2 or >40% LA area (or variable size wall-impinging jet swirling in LA)
Pulmonary venous flow	Normal systolic dominance	Systolic blunting	Systolic flow reversal
Pulmonary hypertension	Not present	May be present	Often present
Continuous wave Doppler	Not dense	Dense, usually parabolic	Dense, early-peaking triangular
Pulse wave mitral Doppler	Dominant A, may be mitral E<A	Variable	Dominant E, never mitral E<A
LV size	Normal	Normal or dilated	Usually dilated
LA size	Normal	Normal or dilated	Usually dilated

*The vena contracta is the narrowest diameter of the jet flow stream that occurs at or just downstream from the orifice. It characteristically has high velocity, laminar flow and is slightly smaller than the anatomical regurgitant orifice due to boundary effects. The cross-sectional area reflects the effective regurgitant orifice area (EROA), which is the narrowest area of actual flow. The diameter of the regurgitant orifice is independent of flow rate and driving pressure (for a fixed orifice). It is estimated from colour flow Doppler. Because of the small values of the width of the vena contracta (usually <1 cm), small errors in measurement can lead to a large percentage error and misjudgement of severity of regurgitation. Hence, the importance of accurate acquisition of primary data and measurement.

**PISA = proximal isovelocity surface area. Aliasing velocity set at 40 cm/s. (See Section 3.2 on continuity equation.)

Based on data from Zoghbi WA, Enriquez-Sarano M, Foster E, et al. Recommendations for evaluation of the severity of native valvular regurgitation with two-dimensional and Doppler echocardiography. J Am Soc Echocardiogr. 2003;16:777–802.

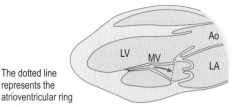

The dotted line represents the atrioventricular ring

Figure 2.11 Prolapse of anterior and posterior mitral valve leaflets.

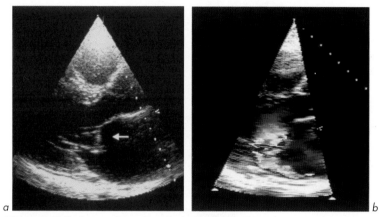

a   b

Figure 2.12 Prolapse of anterior mitral valve leaflet (arrow) on parasternal short-axis view. This leads to an eccentric jet of mitral regurgitation along the posterior wall of left atrium.

MITRAL VALVE PROLAPSE

MV prolapse is a common condition affecting up to 5% of the population (Figs. 2.11, 2.12, 5.10). There is a wide clinical spectrum. It is also known as floppy or billowing MV. It can cause anything from an audible click to severe MR. It may be an isolated finding or associated with other conditions, such as Marfan's syndrome, secundum ASD, Turner's syndrome, Ehlers–Danlos syndrome or other collagen disorders.

The MV leaflets have increased (redundant) tissue and there may be progressive stretching of these and the chordae. People often have atypical non-anginal chest pains and palpitations. There is a risk of endocarditis (antibiotic prophylaxis advice may be given for all dental treatment and surgery, although there is some controversy regarding this and there are country-specific variations in guidance) and complications may develop such as progressive MR, embolization, arrhythmias and sudden death.

There are characteristic M-mode and 2-D echo appearances. The echo diagnosis is made if there is systolic movement of part of either MV leaflet above the plane of the annulus in a long-axis view.

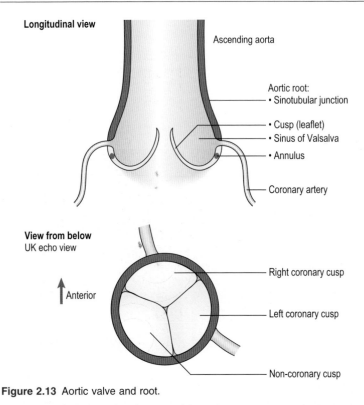

Longitudinal view

Ascending aorta

Aortic root:
• Sinotubular junction

• Cusp (leaflet)
• Sinus of Valsalva
• Annulus

Coronary artery

View from below
UK echo view

Anterior

Right coronary cusp

Left coronary cusp

Non-coronary cusp

Figure 2.13 Aortic valve and root.

2.2 AORTIC VALVE (AV)

The AV is located at the junction of the LV outflow tract and the ascending aorta. The valve usually has 3 cusps (leaflets) attached to an annulus (which is partly fibrous and partly muscular) – one cusp is located on the anterior wall (right cusp), and 2 are located on the posterior wall (left and posterior cusps). Behind each cusp, the aortic wall bulges to form an aortic sinus of Valsalva. The coronary arteries arise from the sinuses (right coronary – anterior sinus, left coronary – left posterior sinus) (Fig. 2.13).

The AV can be studied by M-mode, 2-D and Doppler techniques. In the parasternal long-axis view, the AV cusps open and close on 2-D imaging and an M-mode can be obtained (Figs. 1.13b, 2.14).

The aortic cusps form a central closure line in diastole. In systole, the cusps open and close again at end-systole when the aortic pressure exceeds the LV pressure, to form a parallelogram shape. Rarely, echoes from the left coronary cusp may be seen within the parallelogram. The LV ejection time can be measured from the point of cusp opening to cusp closing. It is possible to measure aortic root diameter and LA diameter from this M-mode image.

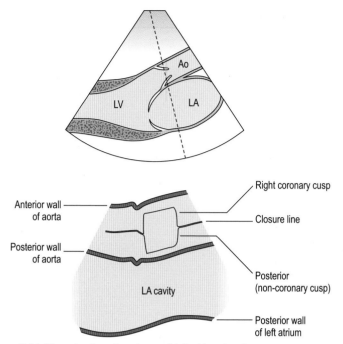

Figure 2.14 M-mode at aortic valve and left atrium level.

A number of abnormal patterns of AV movement on M-mode are seen (Fig. 2.15):

- *Bicuspid AV*. This congenital abnormality affects 1–2% of the population and results in cusps that separate normally but usually have an eccentric closure line that may lie anteriorly or posteriorly. (Note that in up to 15% of cases, the closure line is central.) An eccentric closure line may alternatively be caused in a tricuspid AV when there is a subaortic VSD and prolapse of the right coronary cusp. 2-D echo (especially the parasternal short-axis view at the AV level) can help to differentiate between a bicuspid and a tricuspid AV, but this can be difficult if the valve is heavily calcified. Bicuspid AV is an important cause of AS and may co-exist with other congenital abnormalities such as coarctation of the aorta.
- *Calcific AS*. There are dense echoes usually throughout systole and diastole, which may make cusp movement difficult to see.
- *Vegetations*. These can usually be seen by echo if they are 2 mm or more in diameter (transoesophageal echocardiography [TOE] may visualize smaller vegetations [Section 5.1]). These usually give multiple echoes in diastole, but if large can also be seen during systole. Distinction from calcific AS can be difficult on M-mode.
- *Fibromuscular ring (subaortic stenosis)*. There is immediate systolic closure of the AV, usually best seen on the right coronary cusp. The

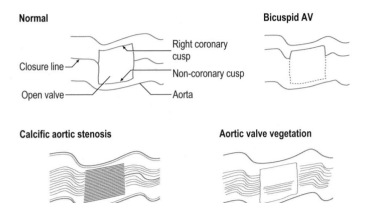

Normal

Closure line

Open valve

Right coronary cusp

Non-coronary cusp

Aorta

Bicuspid AV

Calcific aortic stenosis

Aortic valve vegetation

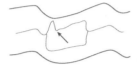

Subaortic stenosis – fibromuscular ring

HCM

Aortic prosthesis (St Jude)

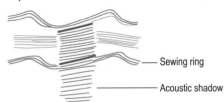

Sewing ring

Acoustic shadow

Figure 2.15 Aortic valve M-mode patterns.

valve cusp may not return to its full open position during systole. This is usually best seen on 2-D echo.

- *HCM.* Premature closure of the AV occurs in mid-systole due to LVOTO when the IVS and AMVL meet.
- *Prosthetic (artificial) AV.* Different types of valve produce various appearances, related to the sewing ring, ball or discs (Chapter 6).

AORTIC STENOSIS (AS)

AS may occur at 3 levels – valvular, subvalvular or supravalvular.

Valvular AS. Has 3 main causes:
1. Rheumatic heart disease. Rarely occurs in isolation (2%) and usually in association with mitral disease.

2. Calcific (degenerative) AS associated with increasing age. The most common cause in Western countries. Minor thickening of the AV is found in 20% of people aged >65 years and 40% of people aged >75 years. This can progress. Aortic sclerosis is a term that should be avoided as it implies a benign course, which is not always correct.

3. Congenital bicuspid valve (1–2% of the population) – a bicuspid AV is found in 40% of middle-aged people with AS and 80% of elderly people with AS.

Subvalvular AS. This is caused by obstruction proximal to the AV:
1. Subaortic membrane
2. HCM
3. Tunnel subaortic obstruction
4. Upper septal bulge. This is due to fibrosis and hypertrophy, usually in elderly people. It unusually may cause obstruction.

Supravalvular AS. This occurs in some congenital conditions such as Williams syndrome (which includes hypercalcaemia, developmental delay, learning disabilities and cognitive challenges).

Clinical evidence of severe AS

Echo is an excellent and important method of assessing the degree of severity of AS, but remember there are important **clinical** features that might suggest severe AS.

A mnemonic may help you to remember these features – symptoms and signs – which can be predicted from simple physiology:

Symptoms of severe AS – 5 A's

1. **A**symptomatic – AS is often an incidental finding.
2. **A**ngina – even with normal coronary arteries. Due to increased LV oxygen demand, due to raised wall stress or LVH and supply – demand imbalance.
3. **A**rrhythmia – causing palpitations.
4. **A**ttacks of unconsciousness, i.e. syncope. May be due to arrhythmia or LVOTO but is not always related to pressure gradient across the valve.
5. '**A**sthma' (cardiac), i.e. breathlessness, due to raised LV diastolic pressure. Not true asthma. Pulmonary oedema (which can cause bronchospasm and wheezing) due to LV failure in severe AS is a very serious – often fatal – occurrence, taking place late in the disease process.

Signs of severe AS – 4 S's

1. **S**low-rising pulse – due to LVOTO.
2. **S**ystolic blood pressure (BP) low – due to LVOTO.

3. Sustained apex beat – due to LVH from pressure overload. The apex is not displaced as the external heart size does not increase – the heart hypertrophies 'inwards'.

4. Second heart sound abnormalities – these range from soft, narrow-split, single (only P_2 heard), reversed split (A_2–P_2 splitting paradoxically shorter in inspiration) based on severity of AS, effect upon LV ejection time and mobility of aortic cusps.

One very important fact to remember: The severity of AS is **NOT** related to the loudness of the murmur. Turbulent flow across a mildly narrowed valve can cause a very loud murmur. Conversely, a very severely narrowed valve may cause marked restriction to blood flow and may be associated with only a very soft murmur.

Echo features of AS

The **M-mode** features of AS have been mentioned. On **2-D echo** using parasternal long- and short-axis views and apical 5-chamber views:

1. The cusps may be thickened, calcified, have reduced motion or may 'dome' (the latter is usually diagnostic of AS).

2. There may be LVH due to pressure overload.

3. LV dilatation occurs if heart failure has developed (usually a poor prognostic feature).

4. Post-stenotic dilatation of the aorta may be seen.

Doppler is most useful in determining the severity of AS by estimating the pressure gradient across the AV (Fig. 2.16). Valve area can be calculated using the continuity equation (Chapter 3).

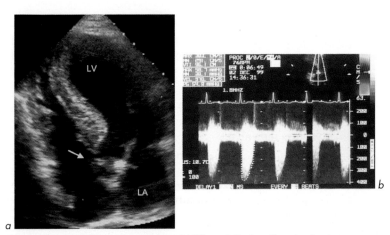

Figure 2.16 Calcific aortic stenosis. **(a)** The calcified aortic valve is shown (arrow) in this apical 5-chamber view. **(b)** Continuous Doppler shows a peak velocity of 3.7 m/s (peak gradient of 54 mmHg).

Table 2.3 Features of varying degrees of aortic stenosis (AS) – based upon EAE/ASE guidelines

	Valve area (cm²)	Indexed valve area (corrected for BSA) (cm²/m²)		
Normal	3.0–4.0	1.8–2.4		
Mild	1.6–2.9	>0.85		
Moderate	1.0–1.5	0.6–0.85		
Severe	<1.0*	<0.6		
	Peak velocity (m/s)	Velocity ratio[†]	Peak gradient (mmHg)	Mean gradient (mmHg)
Normal	1.0–2.5**	1.0	<10	<10
Mild	2.6–2.9	>0.5	27–35	<20[‡] (<30[§])
Moderate	3.0–4.0	0.25–0.5	36–64	20–40[‡] (30–50[§])
Severe	>4.0	<0.25	>64	>40[‡] (>50[§])

*Some authorities use <0.75 cm² as severe. **≤2.5 m/s may indicate aortic sclerosis. [†]Ratio of left ventricular outflow tract peak velocity to AV peak velocity. [‡]AHA/ACC guidance; [§]ESC guidance. Based on data from Baumgartner H, Hung J, Bermejo J, et al. Echocardiographic assessment of valve stenosis: EAE/ASE recommendations for clinical practice. Eur J Echocardiogr. 2009;10:1-25.

Severity of AS correlates with valve area, peak velocity, peak pressure gradient and mean pressure gradient (often more accurate than peak) (see Table 2.3).

The AV pressure gradients depend on cardiac output. They can be overestimated in high-output states (e.g. anaemia) and underestimated in low-output states (e.g. systolic heart failure). The continuity equation helps in this case (Section 3.2).

Surgical intervention (valve replacement)

This is indicated in:
- Severe AS (maximum gradient >64 mmHg, mean gradient >40 mmHg)
- AS of lesser extent with symptoms (e.g. syncope)
- Severe AS with LV systolic dysfunction
- Severe/moderate AS at other cardiac surgery (e.g. coronary bypass)
- Asymptomatic severe AS with expected high exertion or pregnancy.

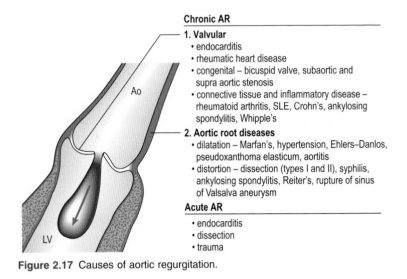

Chronic AR

1. Valvular
- endocarditis
- rheumatic heart disease
- congenital – bicuspid valve, subaortic and supra aortic stenosis
- connective tissue and inflammatory disease – rheumatoid arthritis, SLE, Crohn's, ankylosing spondylitis, Whipple's

2. Aortic root diseases
- dilatation – Marfan's, hypertension, Ehlers–Danlos, pseudoxanthoma elasticum, aortitis
- distortion – dissection (types I and II), syphilis, ankylosing spondylitis, Reiter's, rupture of sinus of Valsalva aneurysm

Acute AR
- endocarditis
- dissection
- trauma

Figure 2.17 Causes of aortic regurgitation.

AORTIC REGURGITATION (AR)

This is leakage of blood from the aorta into the LV during diastole (Fig. 2.17).

Echo diagnosis of AR

All the echo modalities are useful in diagnosis and evaluation. Doppler and colour flow mapping are especially helpful. M-mode and 2-D echo cannot directly diagnose AR but may indicate underlying causes (e.g. dilated aortic root, bicuspid AV) and aid in the assessment of the effects of AR (e.g. LV dilatation).

M-mode may show:
- Vegetations on AV
- Fluttering of AV cusps in diastole (e.g. rupture due to endocarditis or degeneration)
- Eccentric closure line of bicuspid valve
- Dilatation of aortic root
- Fluttering of anterior MV leaflet
- Premature opening of AV because of raised left ventricular end-diastolic pressure (LVEDP) and premature closure of MV. Both suggest severe AR
- Dilatation of LV cavity due to volume overload
- Exaggerated septal and posterior wall of LV wall motion (exaggerated septal early dip strongly suggests AR).

2-D echo may show:
- LV dilatation – correlates with severity of AR
- Abnormal leaflets (bicuspid, rheumatic)

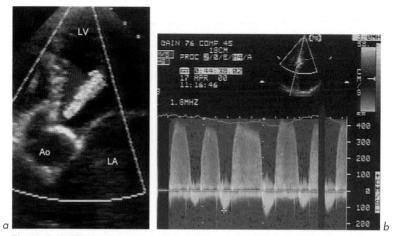

a   b

Figure 2.18 Mild aortic regurgitation. **(a)** Zoomed apical 5-chamber view showing a narrow jet extending a short distance into LV cavity on colour flow mapping. **(b)** Continuous wave Doppler. Note beat-to-beat variation since subject is in atrial fibrillation.

- Vegetations
- Dilated aortic root
- Proximal aortic dissection
- Abnormal indentation of the anterior MV leaflet
- Abnormal interventricular septal motion.

Doppler

This is useful both for detecting AR and assessing its severity. Colour flow mapping is helpful. The jet of AR can be seen entering the LV cavity on a number of views such as parasternal long-axis and apical 5-chamber. Pulsed Doppler can be used in the apical 5-chamber view with the sample volume just proximal to the AV. AR can be detected as a signal above the baseline (towards the transducer) but since AR velocity is usually high (>2 m/s) aliasing will occur. Continuous wave Doppler is then useful and the signal is seen above the baseline (Fig. 2.18).

There are 2 possible complicating factors:

1. The AR jet may be missed, especially if eccentric. Colour flow mapping can detect the jet and aid in placing the pulse wave sample volume, which can be moved around the entire LVOT in a number of different views.

2. The AR jet may be difficult to differentiate from a high-velocity jet of MS, especially in apical 5-chamber view (the 2 often co-exist!).

Colour flow mapping can confirm which or if both conditions are present and pulsed Doppler is used to map the LVOT and MV areas separately. Continuous Doppler of AR shows a velocity signal starting

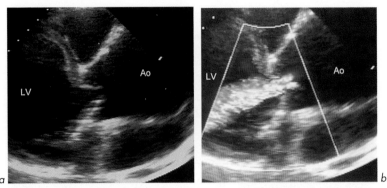

Figure 2.19 Severe aortic regurgitation due to aneurysmal dilatation of aortic root. Parasternal long-axis views.

early in and lasting throughout diastole with a high peak velocity (>2 m/s). MS produces a mid-diastolic velocity signal, usually with a peak velocity of <2 m/s.

Assessing the severity of AR

As with MR, assessing severity of AR is not straightforward. A number of echo criteria are used:

1. Effects on the LV

2. The volume of blood regurgitating across the valve

3. The rate of fall of the pressure gradient between the aorta and LV.

M-mode and 2-D echo show LV dilatation with severe AR. Progressive dilatation with symptoms or left ventricular end-systolic diameter (LVESD) in excess of 5.5 cm are indications for surgical intervention.

Doppler is quite good at indicating severe AR (Fig. 2.19) but not so good at distinguishing between mild and moderate AR.

Using **pulsed wave Doppler**, the sample volume can be placed in various positions within the LV cavity to give a semi-quantitative idea of severity by seeing how far into the LV cavity the AR jet reaches. As a broad guide, mild AR remains within the area of the AV, moderate AR remains between the left ventricular outflow tract (LVOT) and the level of the MV above papillary muscle level and severe AR extends to the LV apex.

This only gives a rough approximation – a narrow jet of mild AR may extend deep into the LV cavity, whilst a severe broad jet of AR may be eccentrically angled and not extend far into the LV.

Using **colour flow mapping**, the width of the AR jet immediately below the AV indicates severity. This relates to the area of failed valvular apposition (the regurgitant orifice). A jet width >60% of aortic width at cusp level is usually severe. A frozen image of AR can be taken and planimetry used to estimate the cross-sectional area of the jet. The length of the AR jet into the LV cavity on apical 5-chamber view can also indicate severity (longer jet – more severe AR).

With **continuous wave Doppler**, the slope of the deceleration rate of the Doppler signal of AR can give an indication of severity as can the intensity of the signal (more intense – more severe AR). The basis for this is described in Chapter 3. Diastolic flow reversal in the aortic arch also suggests severe AR.

As with acute-onset MR, these echo features of severe AR may not all be present in *acute* AR (e.g. due to endocarditis that has destroyed the valve, dissection of the ascending aorta or trauma). The LV cavity has not had time to dilate and so even a relatively small-volume high-velocity jet of AR into the LV may cause a rise in LVEDP, which causes breathlessness and may cause pulmonary oedema.

ASE guidelines to assess severity of AR are shown in Table 2.4.

Table 2.4 Severity of aortic regurgitation (AR) – based upon ASE guidelines

	Mild	Moderate	Severe
Jet width/LVOT	<25%	25–64%	>65%
Vena contracta width*	<0.3 cm	0.3–0.6 cm	>0.6 cm
Jet density – continuous wave Doppler	Incomplete or faint	Dense	Dense
Pressure half-time	Slow >500 ms	Medium 200–500 ms	Steep <200 ms
Deceleration	<2 m/s²	2–3 m/s²	>3 m/s²
Regurgitant volume/beat	<30 mL	30–59 mL	>60 mL
Regurgitant fraction	<30%	30–49%	>50%
Regurgitant orifice area	<0.1 cm²	0.1–0.29 cm²	>0.3 cm²
Aortic flow reversal	Minimal, brief early diastolic	Intermediate	Prominent, pan-diastolic
LV size	Normal	Normal or dilated	Usually dilated

*The vena contracta is the narrowest diameter of the flow stream. It reflects the diameter of the regurgitant orifice and is independent of flow rate and driving pressure. See Table 2.1.

Based on data from Zoghbi AW, Enriquez-Sarano M, Foster E, et al. Recommendations for evaluation of the severity of native valvular regurgitation with two-dimensional and Doppler echocardiography. J Am Soc Echocardiogr. 2003;16:777–802.

Indications for surgery in AR

The timing of surgical repair of chronic AR is a difficult decision. Progressive LV dilatation and/or impairment can indicate the need for valve replacement. This is particularly true if symptoms develop (e.g. breathlessness, reduced exercise capacity). The main indications are:

- Symptomatic severe AR with or without LV systolic dysfunction
- Asymptomatic severe AR with LV systolic dysfunction or dilatation, particularly if progressive (ejection fraction (EF) <50%, LVESD >55 mm).

In acute AR, urgent surgery is often based clinically upon the degree of haemodynamic compromise and the underlying cause (e.g. dissection of the aorta).

2.3 TRICUSPID VALVE (TV)

TRICUSPID STENOSIS (TS)

Abnormalities of the TV should not be overlooked. It is not unknown for rheumatic MS to be surgically repaired, only for it to be subsequently discovered that the diagnosis of co-existent rheumatic TS was not made preoperatively!

The TV is structurally similar to the MV in having:

- Leaflets – the TV has 3, as its name suggests, unlike the 2 of the MV
- Chordae attached to papillary muscles (subvalvular apparatus)
- An annulus or valve ring – which has a larger area than that of the MV, normal TV area 5–8 cm^2.

The most common cause of TS is rheumatic heart disease. There is nearly always co-existent MS. TS occurs about 10 times less commonly. Other rare causes of TS include carcinoid syndrome (excessive secretion of 5-hydroxytryptamine [5-HT] usually from a malignant intra-abdominal tumour causes TS, asthma, flushing, etc.; often associated with TR); RA tumours (e.g. myxoma causing obstruction); obstruction of RV inflow tract (rare – vegetations, extracardiac tumours, pericardial constriction); congenital (Ebstein's anomaly, Chapter 6) or right-sided endocarditis (intravenous drug abusers or following cannulation of veins).

M-mode and 2-D echo findings are analogous to MS:

- Thick and/or calcified leaflets
- Restricted leaflet motion
- Doming of one or more leaflets in diastole (especially the anterior leaflet).

In rheumatic disease, the leaflets are thick and the tips are fused. In carcinoid, the tips tend to be separate and mobile. In severe TS, the RA and IVC are dilated.

Doppler findings are similar to MS. Trans-tricuspid flow is best measured with pulsed Doppler in the apical 4-chamber view with the sample volume in the RV immediately below the TV. There is increased flow velocity in diastole. Evaluation of severity is rarely needed in clinical practice, but is by similar principles as indicated for MS (diastolic pressure gradient and valve area). Severe TS is usually associated with a peak gradient of 3–10 mmHg and a mean gradient >5 mmHg, with a valve area ≤1.0 cm^2.

The pressure half-time equation used for MS (Section 3.1) is empirical and the constant should not be applied to TS.

TRICUSPID REGURGITATION (TR) (Figs. 2.20, 2.21)

Virtually every TV shows some TR during its normal function. This fact allows the use of Doppler echo to estimate PASP (Section 3.1).

Causes of TR are similar to MR – the most common causes are secondary to RV dilatation (dilating the TV annulus), and primary causes include disease of the leaflets and/or the subvalvular apparatus.

Secondary causes – most common

- Pulmonary hypertension (PHT)
- Pulmonary valve disease
- Cor pulmonale (right heart failure associated with lung disease such as emphysema)
- Ischaemic heart disease

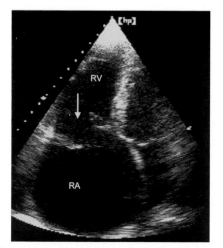

Figure 2.20 Prolapse of the tricuspid valve (apical 4-chamber view).

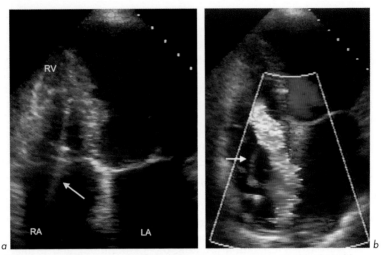

Figure 2.21 Pacing wire. **(a)** The wire (arrow) passes through the tricuspid valve from right atrium to right ventricle. **(b)** Associated with an eccentric jet of tricuspid regurgitation. Apical 4-chamber views.

- Cardiomyopathies
- Volume overload (e.g. ASD, VSD)
- Interference with normal valve closure (e.g. pacing lead).

Primary causes

- Infective endocarditis
- Rheumatic heart disease
- Carcinoid
- Chordal rupture
- Papillary muscle dysfunction
- TV prolapse
- Connective tissue diseases
- Rheumatoid arthritis
- Congenital, e.g. Ebstein's anomaly.

Echo assessment of TR severity is best achieved by Doppler as with MR. More severe TR is associated with a broad, high-intensity jet filling the RA. There is associated retrograde systolic flow in the vena cava and hepatic vein.

2.4 PULMONARY VALVE (PV)

The PV has 3 leaflets and sits at the junction of the right ventricular outflow tract (RVOT) and the main pulmonary artery (PA).

Table 2.5 Severity of pulmonary stenosis – based upon EAE/ASE guidelines

Severity of PS	Peak velocity (m/s)	Peak gradient (mmHg)	Valve area (cm²)
Mild	<3	<36	>1.0
Moderate	3.0–4.0	36–64	0.5–1.0
Severe	>4.0	>64	<0.5

Based on data from Baumgartner H, Hung J, Bermejo J, et al. Echocardiographic assessment of valve stenosis: EAE/ASE recommendations for clinical practice. Eur J Echocardiogr. 2009;10:1-25.

PULMONARY STENOSIS (PS)

As with AS, PS may be valvular, supravalvular (peripheral) or subvalvular (infundibular).

Valvular PS may be congenital (most common – isolated, or as part of another syndrome, e.g. Noonan's, tetralogy of Fallot or rubella) or acquired (rheumatic, carcinoid).

Assessment of severity is along similar principles to AS (see Table 2.5). **2-D echo** may show thickened, calcified leaflets, doming of the valve leaflets in systole and restricted motion. There may be post-stenotic dilatation of the PA or its branches and RV hypertrophy or dilatation due to pressure overload.

The normal peak velocity across the valve is 1.0 m/s and valve area is 3–5 cm². The peak gradient across the valve can be estimated by **Doppler**. This correlates with estimated valve area.

There may be few symptoms and quite severe PS may be well tolerated into adult life.

Supravalvular PS can be due to stenosis of the main PA or any of its branches distal to the PV (e.g. rubella – often with PDA or infantile hypercalcaemia – with supra-aortic stenosis). It may be iatrogenic – post-surgical banding of the PA, which is performed in some left-to-right shunts as a temporary measure to protect the pulmonary circulation.

One or more discrete shelf-like bands may be seen in the PA on 2-D echo. A long stenotic tapering tunnel area may be seen distal to the PV. The increase in Doppler velocity detected by pulsed wave Doppler is distal to and not at the level of the PV.

Subvalvular PS is most commonly congenital – rarely isolated, usually in association with valvular stenosis, VSD, tetralogy of Fallot and transposition of the great arteries. May also occur in hypertrophic cardiomyopathies. Acquired causes, e.g. tumours, are very rare.

A muscular band and/or narrowing of the subvalvular area are seen. Usually there is no post-stenotic dilatation. Using pulsed wave

Doppler, it can be seen that the increase in velocity occurs in the RVOT below the level of the PV.

PULMONARY REGURGITATION (PR)

Secondary causes – most common

- Dilatation of the PA – PHT, Marfan's syndrome.

Primary causes

- Infective endocarditis
- Rheumatic heart disease
- Carcinoid
- Congenital (e.g. absence or malformation of PV leaflets, or following surgery for tetralogy of Fallot)
- Iatrogenic (e.g. post-valvotomy or catheter-induced at angiography)
- Syphilis.

M-mode and 2-D echo cannot detect PR directly but can show some evidence of the underlying cause and the effect. There may be evidence of:
- PHT – dilated RV, dilated PA, abnormal IVS motion (behaves as though it 'belongs' to the RV rather than LV – 'right ventricularization' of IVS)
- Dilated PA – the diameter can be measured usually in parasternal short-axis view at AV level
- Vegetation on the valve in endocarditis
- Thick immobile PV leaflets in rheumatic heart disease or carcinoid
- Absent valve leaflets (congenital)
- PA aneurysm.

Doppler techniques show PR and help to assess severity, as with AR. Doppler indicators of severe PR are:
- Colour flow – the regurgitant jet is visualized directly. Severity is indicated by the width of the jet at valve level, how far into RV it extends and the area of the jet by planimetry
- Pulsed wave Doppler – the distance between the PV and the level at which PR is detected can be determined. A jet at the lower infundibular region is severe
- Increased intensity of the Doppler signal
- Increased slope of the Doppler signal (deceleration time; DT).

DOPPLER – VELOCITIES AND PRESSURES

3.1 SPECIAL USES OF DOPPLER

The Doppler effect (Fig. 3.1), described by the Austrian physicist and mathematician Christian Johann Doppler in 1842, is a change in the frequency of sound, light or other waves caused by the motion of the source or the observer. An example is the change in the sound of an ambulance siren as it approaches (higher pitch) and then passes (lower pitch) an observer. The change is due to compression and rarefaction of sound waves. There is a direct relationship between the relative velocity of the sound source and the observer and the change in pitch.

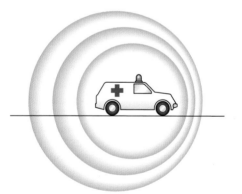

Figure 3.1 Doppler effect.

MEASURING BLOOD VELOCITY AND PRESSURE GRADIENTS

The Doppler effect can be used to examine the direction and velocity of blood flow in blood vessels and within the heart. Ultrasound waves of a known frequency (usually around 2 MHz) are transmitted from the transducer and are reflected by moving blood back towards the transducer, which also acts as an ultrasound receiver. If the blood

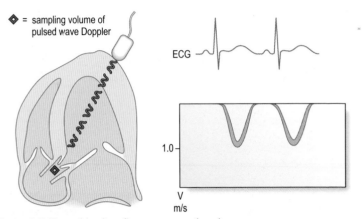

◆ = sampling volume of
pulsed wave Doppler

ECG

1.0

V
m/s

Figure 3.2 Normal laminar flow across aortic valve.

is moving towards the transducer, the frequency of the ultrasound signal increases and vice versa. This can be used by computer analysis to derive haemodynamic information such as the nature and severity of valvular abnormalities (e.g. valvular stenosis) since it is possible to relate velocity to pressure difference (also referred to as pressure gradient) by a simple equation (see the *Bernoulli equation* below). Doppler can also detect the presence of valvular regurgitation and give an indication of its severity. This information can complement the anatomical information provided by M-mode and 2-D echo techniques. The Doppler-measured flow patterns and velocities across the heart valves can be displayed graphically against time on the monitor of the echo machine or printed on paper. By convention, velocities towards the transducer are displayed above the line and those away from it below the line. The normal flow patterns for the aortic and mitral valves are shown (Figs. 3.2, 3.3).

This is a graph of velocity against time, but it also gives a densitometric dimension, since the density of any spot is related to the strength of the reflected signal, which relates to the number of reflecting red blood cells moving at that velocity. In normal situations where blood flow is laminar (smooth), most of the blood cells travel at about the same velocity, accelerating and decelerating together (Fig. 3.4). The Doppler pattern then has an outline form with very few cells travelling at other velocities at a given time. When there is turbulence of flow, e.g. due to a narrowed valve, there is a wide distribution of blood cell velocities, and the Doppler signal is 'filled in'.

Note that for aortic flow, the blood is moving away from the transducer placed at the cardiac apex and the Doppler signal is displayed below the baseline. The opposite is true for mitral flow, which is predominantly towards the apex.

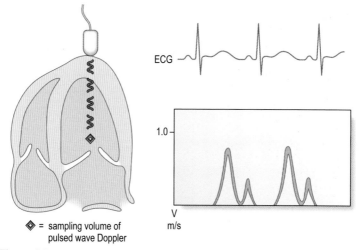

= sampling volume of
pulsed wave Doppler

Figure 3.3 Normal laminar flow across mitral valve.

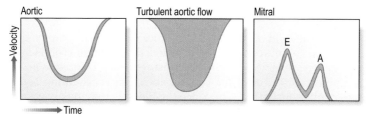

Figure 3.4 Normal laminar pulsed wave Doppler patterns and turbulent aortic flow pattern.

Table 3.1 Doppler velocities in healthy adults and children

Valve	Peak (m/s)	Range (m/s)
AV/aorta	1.3	0.9–1.7
LV	0.9	0.7–1.1
MV	0.9	0.6–1.3
TV	0.5	0.3–0.7
PV/PA	0.75	0.5–1.0

The usual peak Doppler velocities in healthy adults and children are shown in Table 3.1. Doppler can be used to measure velocities and estimate pressure gradients across narrowed (stenosed) valves.

The normal stroke volume in a resting adult is approximately 70 mL. This volume of blood passes across the AV with each ventricular systole, at a blood velocity of approximately 1 m/s. If the

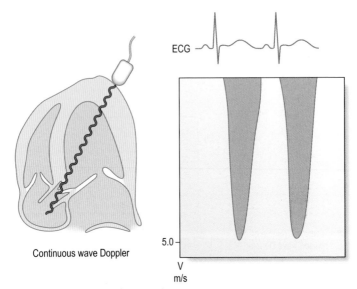

ECG

5.0

Continuous wave Doppler

V
m/s

Figure 3.5 Doppler – aortic stenosis.

AV is stenosed, with a smaller valve orifice cross-sectional area, then for the same volume of blood to be ejected, the blood must accelerate, and this increase in velocity can be measured using Doppler with the ultrasound transducer at the cardiac apex and transmitting sound waves continuously (Fig. 3.5). Since the blood is moving away from the echo transducer, the Doppler velocity signal is below the baseline. In this case, the peak blood velocity across the AV is 5 m/s.

There is a direct and simple relationship between the velocity of blood across a narrowing (stenosis) and the pressure gradient (drop) across the narrowing (not the absolute pressure). This is known as the simplified *Bernoulli equation*:

$$\Delta P = 4V^2$$

where ΔP is the pressure gradient (in mmHg) and V is the peak blood velocity (in m/s) measured by Doppler across the narrowing. In the example shown of AS (Fig. 3.5), the peak Doppler velocity is 5 m/s, which gives an estimated AV gradient of 100 mmHg (severe AS).

USES AND LIMITATIONS OF DOPPLER

The main advantage of Doppler is that it allows accurate haemodynamic measurements to be made non-invasively. The pressure gradient measured has the added advantage of being a true physiological instantaneous gradient (i.e. a gradient that exists in real-time) unlike the peak-to-peak pressure gradient that is calculated

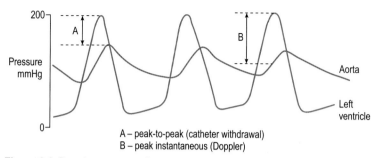

A – peak-to-peak (catheter withdrawal)
B – peak instantaneous (Doppler)

Figure 3.6 Doppler measures instantaneous pressure gradient.

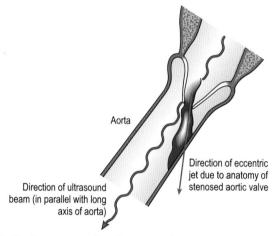

Figure 3.7 Continuous wave Doppler may underestimate the velocity of an eccentric jet.

from most cardiac catheterization studies, since the peak LV pressure and peak aortic pressure do not occur simultaneously (Fig. 3.6).

An equation has been derived that approximately relates peak-to-peak aortic pressure gradient (from catheterization) to peak instantaneous Doppler gradient:

$$\text{Peak-to-peak gradient} \approx (0.84 \times \text{peak Doppler gradient}) - 14 \text{ mmHg}$$

The main limitation of using the Doppler technique is that blood velocity is a vector (it has direction). Therefore, it is essential that the ultrasound beam is lined up in parallel with the direction of blood flow, otherwise the peak velocity (and consequently the valve pressure gradient) will be underestimated. This can be especially difficult when the direction of the blood flow jet is eccentric due to the anatomy of the stenosed valve (Fig. 3.7).

Another limitation with pulsed wave Doppler is that it can only examine blood of velocity of less than 2 m/s. Beyond that, an

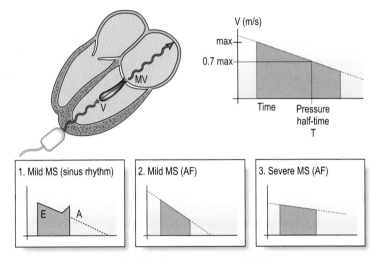

Figure 3.8 Mitral stenosis – Doppler assessment of valve area.

effect known as aliasing occurs and continuous Doppler must be used.

MITRAL STENOSIS

The velocity of blood across the healthy MV is approximately 0.9 m/s. In the presence of MS, blood velocity across the valve increases (Fig. 3.8). This can be measured by continuous wave Doppler and an assessment made of severity of valve stenosis and of valve area.

This is done by looking at the way the pressure across the MV varies with time as blood flows across it. If blood flows across a normal valve, there would be a rapid peak of high-velocity blood and the velocity then falls away quickly as the pressures between LA and LV equalize. In a stenosed valve, the peak in velocity is higher, but the time taken for the pressure gradient to fall away is prolonged, and the more severe the stenosis the more slowly the pressure falls away (remember to think of it as the pressure gradient being maintained for a longer period to push blood across a narrowed valve).

It has been found that the area of the mitral valve (A_{MV}) and the time taken for the pressure gradient to fall away to half its initial peak value (T) are approximately inversely proportional to each other.

If A_{MV} is measured in cm^2 and T in milliseconds, the constant has been found empirically to be equal to 220:

$$A_{MV} = \frac{220}{T}$$

So to estimate A_{MV}, it is sufficient to measure T. Doppler does not measure pressure gradient directly, but measures velocity; pressure gradient is derived from the simplified Bernoulli equation. That means that the pressure gradient will have fallen to half its peak value when the velocity has fallen to $1/\sqrt{2}$ of its peak value, i.e. to 0.7 of its peak value.

Measurement of the time T taken for peak blood velocity to reach 0.7 of its value (equivalent to pressure gradient reaching half its value) is called the **pressure half-time** and a good approximation of A_{MV} is:

$$A_{MV} = \frac{220}{\text{Pressure half-time}}$$

Many echo machines have software packages that allow measurement of pressure half-time and estimation of MV area. It is less accurate for very low pressure half-time.

In many cases of severe MS, the rhythm is AF and there is no second A-wave peak of velocity of the transmitral flow (which is caused by atrial contraction). In this situation, the slope of the top of the Doppler velocity signal can be measured to calculate MV area. Since the heart rate and duration of systole and diastole vary from beat to beat in AF, it is ideal to measure several beats to take the mean value of MV area. When the rhythm is normal sinus rhythm, the slope of the top of the early phase of transmitral flow (E-wave) is taken, and the A-wave is ignored.

The technique should not be used to determine the severity of TS as the constant is not the same.

Mean gradients (rather than peak gradients) can also be helpful in assessing the severity of valvular stenosis (e.g. AS, MS). The mean gradient is derived from the velocity at all time points during blood flow. In practical terms, one traces around the Doppler spectrum envelope and the mean gradient is calculated by the computer of the echo machine.

SEVERITY OF AORTIC REGURGITATION BY CONTINUOUS DOPPLER

As described in Section 2.2, the slope and intensity of the continuous Doppler signal of AR can indicate severity (Fig. 3.9). The greater the slope, the more severe the AR. A steep slope indicates that, as diastole progresses, the pressure gradient across the AV in diastole between the aorta and LV cavity is becoming smaller. The AV is acting less effectively in keeping the 2 areas separated.

Another way to express this is the time taken for the maximum pressure gradient across the AV to drop to half its value – the pressure half-time. The more quickly the pressure difference falls away (or the shorter the pressure half-time), the more severe is the AR (Fig. 3.10).

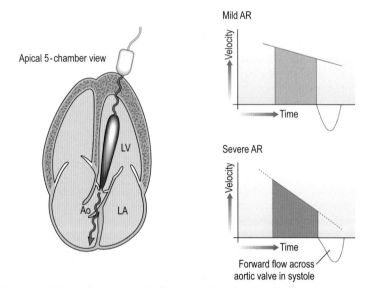

Figure 3.9 Doppler assessment of severity of aortic regurgitation.

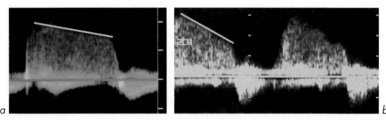

Figure 3.10 Aortic regurgitation. Continuous Doppler patterns showing **(a)** mild aortic regurgitation and **(b)** severe aortic regurgitation.

A correlation has been made between severity and these measurements:

Severity of AR	Deceleration rate of AR (m/s²)	Pressure half-time (ms)
Mild	<2	>500
Moderate	2–3	200–500
Severe	>3	<200

The intensity of the continuous wave Doppler signal also gives a qualitative indication of AR severity. It is more intense in severe AR as a greater volume of blood is moving with a given velocity and reflecting ultrasound to the transducer.

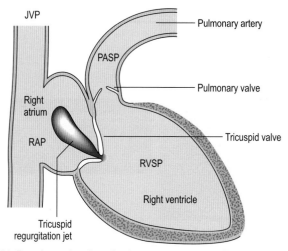

Figure 3.11 Doppler estimation of pulmonary artery systolic pressure from velocity of tricuspid regurgitation.

PA SYSTOLIC PRESSURE FROM TRICUSPID REGURGITATION

Doppler can be used to give a non-invasive measurement of pulmonary artery systolic pressure (PASP) (Fig. 3.11).

This technique takes advantage of the fact that a small degree of TR is found in virtually all normal hearts. The pressure gradient which can be measured using the Bernoulli equation is applied to TR to estimate PASP.

This is how it is done:

1. The aim is to measure PASP. Assuming no PV stenosis, then this is equal to right ventricular systolic pressure (RVSP).

2. RVSP can be easily estimated from the maximum velocity of the TR jet (V_{TR}) using continuous wave Doppler in an apical 4-chamber view (Fig. 3.12). The pressure gradient between the right ventricle and the right atrium across the tricuspid valve (RVSP – right atrial pressure [RAP]) can be estimated by the Bernoulli equation using the maximum V_{TR}:

$$RVSP - RAP = 4V_{TR}^2$$

3. The value of RAP is known – it is equal to the JVP, which can be assessed clinically (in healthy individuals it is usually 0–5 cm of blood, measured from the sternal angle, and 1 cm of blood is almost equal to 1 mmHg).

4. This allows us to estimate that:

$$PASP = RVSP = 4V_{TR}^2 + JVP$$

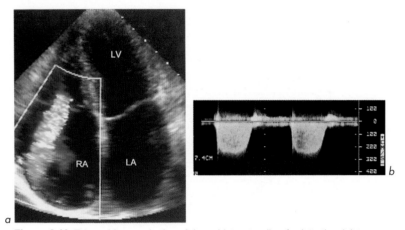

Figure 3.12 Tricuspid regurgitation. A broad jet extending far into the right atrium on colour flow mapping. Continuous Doppler shows a peak velocity of 3.1 m/s, giving an estimated pulmonary artery systolic pressure of 39 mmHg + jugular venous pressure.

If the measured V_{TR} is 2 m/s and the JVP is 0, this gives an approximate PASP of 16 mmHg. The normal value of PASP is up to 25 mmHg.

3.2 CONTINUITY EQUATION

The *continuity equation* is powerful and is used in several situations in echo. It is based upon the principle of the conservation of mass. In the case of a closed system such as the circulation, blood cannot be created or destroyed. The continuity equation can be used to:
- Assess severity of valvular stenosis
- Give an estimate of blood flow and volumes, for example, to measure cardiac output and the size of a shunt (in congenital heart disease)
- Assess severity of valvular regurgitation.

Assessment of severity of AS

In some situations, the Doppler-estimated peak velocity (and hence pressure gradient) across a valve is not a true indication of the severity of valvular stenosis. An example is AS in the presence of LV systolic impairment. This may arise either as a result of long-standing AS that has caused LV impairment, or of AS co-existing with LV disease, for example, dilated cardiomyopathy or ischaemic heart failure. In this situation, the impaired LV may not be able to generate a high velocity across the AV.

The severity of AS can be assessed by calculating the AV orifice area using the *continuity equation* (Fig. 3.13), the principle of which is

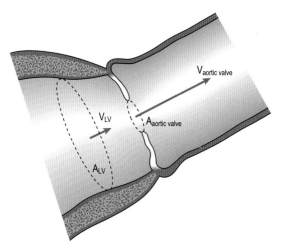

Figure 3.13 Continuity equation.

simple – the volume of blood that leaves the LV in a given time must be the same volume that crosses the AV and enters the aorta.

If a cross-sectional area (A) at a level in the LV is calculated (in cm^2, using M-mode or 2-D measurements) and the velocity of blood (V) at that level measured (in cm/s, using pulsed wave Doppler), the product of area by velocity gives the volume of blood flow at that level (in cm^3/s). As explained above, this volume is the same as that crossing the AV and entering the aorta.

This can be used to measure the area of interest, at AV level ($A_{aortic\ valve}$). The peak velocity across the aortic valve ($V_{aortic\ valve}$) can also be measured by Doppler:

$$A_{aortic\ valve} \times V_{aortic\ valve} = A_{LV} \times V_{LV}$$

$$A_{aortic\ valve} = \frac{A_{LV} \times V_{LV}}{V_{aortic\ valve}}$$

This is not helpful in AS if the peak velocity is <2 m/s. A variation of this method (using the velocity–time integral, VTI) is described below.

ESTIMATION OF BLOOD VOLUMES AND CARDIAC OUTPUT

Although Doppler gives information about blood flow velocity, it can also be used to derive information about blood volumes.

Echo can give an estimate of cardiac output from the left heart:

Cardiac output = stroke volume × heart rate

Stroke volume is derived by echo from a measure known as the 'velocity-time integral' (VTI) (Fig. 3.14). Using pulsed wave or continuous wave Doppler, the area under the velocity–time tracing is the VTI. This can be used to give an indication of blood volume. Aortic VTI can be calculated by the computer of the echo machine as the area under the curve from the pulsed wave or continuous wave Doppler of aortic outflow in the apical 5-chamber view.

VTI is measured in centimetres and is given from peak aortic flow velocity, V_{max} in centimetres/second and aortic ejection time in seconds.

Stroke volume = VTI×cross-sectional area (of aortic valve, CSA)

$$\text{Cross-sectional area (CSA)} = \pi r^2 = \pi\left(\frac{D}{2}\right)^2 \approx \frac{3.142D^2}{4} \approx 0.785D^2$$

$$\text{Stroke volume} \approx \text{VTI} \times 0.785D^2$$

where CSA is the cross-sectional area and D is the AV diameter measured either from the M-mode of the AV tracing or from the parasternal long-axis view measured in the aortic root just above the tips of the aortic cusps.

In practice, it is also possible and more usual to use echo using pulsed wave Doppler to measure the VTI in the LVOT and measure the diameter (D) of the LVOT to give the stroke volume (Fig. 3.14).

Serial measurements of VTI can give non-invasive monitoring of cardiac output, for example in individuals in an intensive care unit (ICU) setting. Cardiac output, or flow in the systemic circulation across the AV, is often abbreviated as Qs (in L/min).

Normal values in adults at rest:
- Stroke volume   70–140 mL/beat
- Cardiac output   4–7 L/min
- Cardiac index*   2.8–4.2 L/min/m^2

(* Cardiac index is cardiac output corrected for BSA.)

A similar method can be used to estimate flow in the pulmonary circulation (Qp). This can be used to estimate the size of a shunt in congenital heart disease (Section 6.4).

Valve area using VTI

The area of a valve (e.g. AV) can also be estimated using the continuity equation and VTI measurements (as an alternative to peak velocity)

a Pulsed wave Doppler – apical 5-chamber (or 3-chamber) view

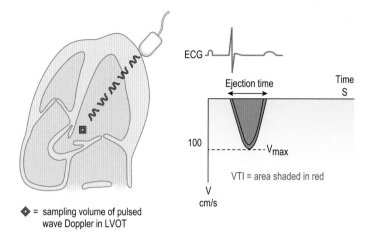

◆ = sampling volume of pulsed
    wave Doppler in LVOT

VTI can be measured by pulsed wave Doppler if V_{max} <2m/s. If V_{max} ≥2m/s, continuous wave Doppler is used

b 2-D echo – parasternal long-axis (zoomed) view to measure LVOT diameter in systole
    (NB use radius [D/2] for area measurements)

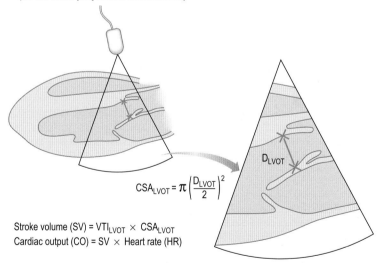

$$CSA_{LVOT} = \pi \left(\frac{D_{LVOT}}{2} \right)^2$$

Stroke volume (SV) = $VTI_{LVOT} \times CSA_{LVOT}$
Cardiac output (CO) = SV × Heart rate (HR)

Figure 3.14 Echo measurement of stroke volume and cardiac output.
(a) Velocity-time integral (VTI) of aortic flow (shaded in red). **(b)** Measurement of cross-sectional area (CSA) of the left ventricular outflow tract (LVOT) (CSA_{LVOT}).

(Fig. 3.15). VTI is measured using pulsed wave Doppler in the LVOT (VTI_{LVOT}) and continuous wave Doppler in the aorta (VTI_{Ao}). The cross-sectional area of the LVOT (CSA_{LVOT}) is also measured from its diameter (D_{LVOT}). The AV area ($A_{aortic\ valve}$) is then given by:

$$A_{aortic\ valve} \times VTI_{Ao} = CSA_{LVOT} \times VTI_{LVOT}$$

$$A_{aortic\ valve} = \frac{CSA_{LVOT} \times VTI_{LVOT}}{VTI_{Ao}}$$

$$CSA_{LVOT} = \pi r^2_{LVOT} = \pi \left(D_{LVOT}/2\right)^2 \approx 0.785 D^2_{LVOT}$$

$$A_{aortic\ valve} \approx \frac{0.785 D^2_{LVOT} \times VTI_{LVOT}}{VTI_{Ao}}$$

A similar method can be used in the RVOT for the PV.

Assessment of valvular regurgitation – understanding the concept of EROA and PISA

Echo and the continuity equation can be used to assess the severity of valvular regurgitation, for example, MR. This gives an estimate of the size of the defect (orifice area) of the regurgitant valve. This is known as the *effective regurgitant orifice area* (EROA). In a normal, non-regurgitant valve, the EROA should ideally be zero. In simple terms, the higher the EROA, the more severe is the regurgitation (more blood can leak through a larger orifice).

EROA is estimated by measuring a value termed the *proximal isovelocity surface area* (PISA). This method is being used increasingly in echo assessment. At first sight, the technique appears complex, but it is worth trying to understand it and to realize that it is a simple concept, based upon the continuity equation and conservation of mass.

Sink analogy

A simple analogy to use is to consider the flow of fluid from a container through a circular hole in the bottom of the container. An example may be water leaving a full sink through an open plug/drain hole, when the hole is opened (Fig. 3.16a).

- As the water approaches the drain hole (orifice), it accelerates and reaches its peak velocity (V_{max}) after it has passed through the hole.
- All the water in the sink at a given distance from the hole has the same velocity, so flow converges around the hole in 3-dimensional (3-D) hemispheric layers/shells (centred around the

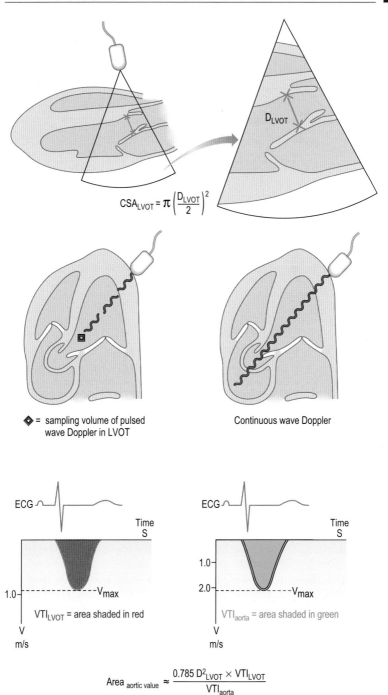

$$CSA_{LVOT} = \pi \left(\frac{D_{LVOT}}{2} \right)^2$$

◆ = sampling volume of pulsed wave Doppler in LVOT

Continuous wave Doppler

VTI_{LVOT} = area shaded in red

VTI_{aorta} = area shaded in green

$$Area_{aortic\ value} \approx \frac{0.785\ D^2_{LVOT} \times VTI_{LVOT}}{VTI_{aorta}}$$

Figure 3.15 Continuity equation. Estimation of aortic valve area using velocity-time integral (VTI) of aortic flow (VTI_{Ao}) and of left ventricular outflow tract (LVOT) (VTI_{LVOT}).

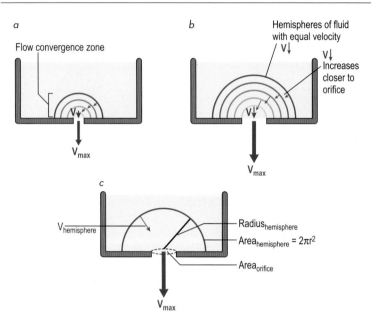

a

Flow convergence zone

V_{max}

b

Hemispheres of fluid with equal velocity

$V\downarrow$

$V\downarrow$ Increases closer to orifice

V_{max}

c

$V_{hemisphere}$

$Radius_{hemisphere}$

$Area_{hemisphere} = 2\pi r^2$

$Area_{orifice}$

V_{max}

From continuity equation:

$$Area_{orifice} \times V_{max} = Area_{hemisphere} \times V_{hemisphere}$$

Figure 3.16 Continuity equation. Sink analogy. **(a)** Flow convergence zone of hemispheric shells (layers) of equal velocity ($V\downarrow$). **(b)** A larger plug/drain hole (orifice) is associated with a larger flow convergence zone and higher peak velocity (V_{max}) through the orifice. **(c)** In a given time, the volume of fluid passing through each hemisphere is equal to the volume passing through the orifice.

hole) of equal velocity. This zone from which the water accelerates is called the *flow convergence zone*.

• The larger the size of the hole, the greater is the distance from which water accelerates towards it (i.e. the larger is the radius of the flow convergence zone) (Fig. 3.16b).

• By using the continuity equation and conservation of mass (the same mass of water entering the hole must leave it in a given time) it is possible to estimate the area of the hole.

• This is the crucial part of the process – to remember that we are dealing with a 3-dimensional system (Fig. 3.16c). The volume of water in a unit time passing through <u>each</u> *hemisphere* towards the hole is:

$$Area_{hemisphere} \times Velocity_{hemisphere} = 2\pi\,(r_{hemisphere})^2 \times Velocity_{hemisphere}$$

• Using the continuity equation, this volume is equal to the volume passing through the hole. So the area of the hole (or orifice area, $A_{orifice}$) is given by:

$$A_{\text{orifice}} \times V_{\text{max}} = \text{Area}_{\text{hemisphere}} \times \text{Velocity}_{\text{hemisphere}}$$

$$A_{\text{orifice}} = \frac{2\pi \, (r_{\text{hemisphere}})^2 \times \text{Velocity}_{\text{hemisphere}}}{V_{\text{max}}}$$

- Thus, if it is possible to measure V_{max} at the orifice and the velocity at a point on the surface of a hemisphere of known radius in the flow convergence zone, then the area of the orifice can be calculated by the continuity equation.

How does this help us with echo and valvular regurgitation, for example, MR?

- In this case, substitute the LV for the sink, the orifice of the regurgitant MV for the plughole and blood for water, in our earlier analogy above (Fig. 3.17a).
- The larger the size of the regurgitant orifice (known as the EROA), the greater the degree of MR and the further back from the orifice the regurgitant blood accelerates (mild regurgitation – smaller flow convergence zone; severe regurgitation – larger flow convergence zone).
- We wish to measure the regurgitant MV orifice area (EROA). From the continuity equation, the volume of blood regurgitating across the MV during systole in each second is given by:

$$EROA \times V_{\text{max}}$$

(V_{max} can be measured by echo using continuous wave Doppler in an apical 4-chamber view.)

- This is equal to the volume of blood reaching the regurgitant MV by passing through each hemisphere of flow convergence in the LV.
- Echo can help to calculate the volume reaching the regurgitant valve in a very elegant way. Colour flow mapping Doppler is used. This can show flow convergence around the regurgitant MV orifice as semicircular rings of different colours (velocities) (Fig. 3.17b).
- Each ring is a 2-D representation of the 3-D hemisphere of a given velocity. The Colour flow mapping gain settings are adjusted in practice to give an aliasing velocity of around 40 cm/s.
- The distance from the MV at which aliasing occurs is displayed on colour flow mapping Doppler as an abrupt colour change. *Blood at this point has the aliasing velocity, which is measured.*
- The distance from the MV orifice to this colour change is the radius of the hemisphere whose velocity is the aliasing velocity. The surface area of this 'aliasing' hemisphere is termed the proximal isovelocity surface area (PISA). PISA is given by:

$$PISA = 2\pi \, (PISA_{\text{radius}})^2$$

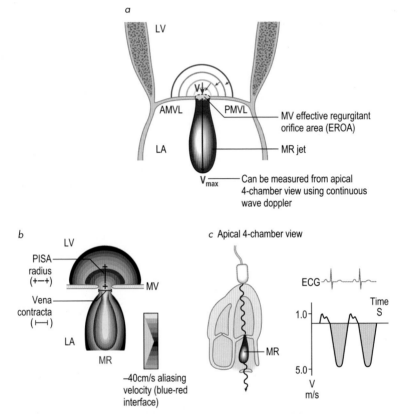

Figure 3.17 Continuity equation. Mitral regurgitation (MR). **(a)** Flow convergence and effective regurgitant orifice area (EROA). **(b)** Schematic representation of colour flow mapping Doppler in MR. The proximal isovelocity surface area (PISA) radius is indicated by the abrupt colour transition from blue to red. The aliasing velocity in this example is 40 cm/s. **(c)** Measurement of MR peak velocity (V_{max}) using continuous wave Doppler in apical 4-chamber view.

- The continuity equation is then used to measure the MV EROA (Fig. 3.17c). This is given from the PISA and $V_{aliasing}$ and the V_{max} of MR measured by continuous wave Doppler, by:

$$EROA \times V_{max} = PISA \times V_{aliasing}$$

$$EROA = \frac{PISA \times V_{aliasing}}{V_{max}}$$

For MR only (not for other valvular regurgitation), a simplification of this PISA technique may be used, termed ***PISA lite***. This assumes that the peak velocity of MR is 500 cm/s (i.e. 5 m/s), which is a reasonable assumption, as the LV–LA pressure difference (= $4V^2$) is often approximately 100 mmHg. If the aliasing velocity is set at 40 cm/s and the radius of the PISA shell is measured, the PISA lite estimate of EROA is given by:

$$\text{EROA} \approx \frac{2\pi\,(\text{PISA}_{\text{radius}})^2 \times 40}{500} \approx \frac{(\text{PISA}_{\text{radius}})^2}{2}$$

The regurgitant volume can also be measured:

$$\text{Regurgitant volume} = \text{EROA} \times \text{VTI}$$

where VTI is the area under the continuous wave Doppler measurement of the MR jet, in the apical 4-chamber view.

This method can be applied to other regurgitant valves. It is a powerful technique and is being used increasingly in the echo assessment of individuals with valvular abnormalities. It has limitations and some advantages and disadvantages.

Advantages of estimating PISA and EROA:
- Provides an estimate of valvular regurgitation that is independent of aetiology, haemodynamic variables and multiple valve abnormalities
- Can be used in central jets (less accurate in eccentric jets)
- Gives a quantitative assessment of severity of regurgitation
- Has acceptable reproducibility.

Disadvantages of estimating PISA and EROA:
- Assumes there is a single, circular, flat regurgitant orifice. If this is not the case, flow convergence will not be hemispheric and PISA cannot be used accurately
- Not useful if there are multiple regurgitant orifices
- Less accurate if regurgitant jet is eccentric
- Errors in PISA measurements are squared
- Systolic changes of regurgitant flow are not taken into account.

HEART FAILURE, MYOCARDIUM AND PERICARDIUM

4.1 HEART FAILURE

There is no ideal definition of heart failure. One definition is of a clinical syndrome caused by an abnormality of the heart which leads to a characteristic pattern of haemodynamic, renal, neural and hormonal responses. A shorter definition is ventricular dysfunction with symptoms.

Echo plays a crucial role when heart failure is suspected (e.g. unexplained breathlessness, clinical signs such as raised venous pressure, basal crackles, third heart sound) to help establish the diagnosis, assess ventricular function and institute correct treatment.

An underlying *cause* of heart failure should always be sought and echo plays an essential role here also (Table 4.1). The most common cause in Western populations is coronary artery disease (CAD). Echo may also reveal a surgically treatable underlying cause (e.g. valvular disease or LV aneurysm). Heart failure may be caused by severe AS (which affects 3% of people aged over 75 years) and the murmur at this stage may be absent.

Major therapeutic advances have been made in the past three decades, including the use of modern diuretics, angiotensin-converting enzyme (ACE) inhibitors, device therapy and cardiac transplantation. This has improved the quality and duration of life of many with heart failure.

Some studies (e.g. Framingham study) have provided epidemiological data on heart failure:

- Incidence is 0.5–1.5% per year, increasing in many countries, because the population is ageing and there has been a reduction in the fatality rate for acute MI
- Almost 50% of patients surviving MI develop heart failure
- Prevalence is 1–3% (above the age of 70 years, it is 5–10%).

The term dilated cardiomyopathy describes large hearts with reduced contractile function in the presence of normal coronary arteries

Table 4.1 Causes of chronic heart failure

Myocardial disease	
Systolic failure	
• Coronary artery disease	Dyskinesia, diffuse dysfunction, aneurysm, inco-ordination, stunning, hibernation
• Cardiomyopathy	Idiopathic – dilated, hypertrophic, restrictive
	Poisons – alcohol, heavy metals, toxins, poisons, doxorubicin, other cardiotoxic drugs
	Myocarditis
	Endocrine (e.g. hypothyroidism)
	Infiltration – amyloid, endomyocardial fibrosis
• Hypertension	
• Drugs	β-Blockers, calcium antagonists, anti-arrhythmic drugs
Diastolic failure	
• Elderly people, ischaemia, hypertrophy	
Arrhythmias	
• Tachycardia	AF, VT, supraventricular tachycardia (SVT)
• Bradycardia	Complete heart block
Pericardial diseases	
Valve dysfunction	
• Pressure overload	Aortic stenosis
• Volume overload	Mitral or aortic regurgitation
• Restricted forward flow	Mitral or aortic stenosis
Shunts	
Extracardiac disease	
'High output' failure	Anaemia, thyrotoxicosis, pregnancy, glomerulonephritis, AV fistula, Paget's disease of bone, beri-beri

Adapted from Kaddoura S, Poole-Wilson A. In: Volta SD, de Luna AB, Braunwald E, eds. Cardiology. McGraw-Hill; 1999:523-533.

(Section 4.4). It is usually of unknown cause. When a cause is established, the term is sometimes preceded by a qualifier, such as alcoholic dilated cardiomyopathy. Hypertension has become a less common cause of heart failure as a consequence of its improved detection and treatment. It remains an important contributory factor to the progression of heart failure and is a risk factor for coronary artery disease.

It is always important to seek the cause of worsening features (decompensation) of heart failure in a previously clinically stable individual. This may lead to symptoms such as breathlessness or signs such as crackles in the chest, raised venous pressure or peripheral oedema. Echo can help in the investigation of the potential causes:

- Non-compliance with medications (e.g. diuretics)
- Myocardial infarction or ischaemia
- Cardiac rhythm change (e.g. AF, VT)
- Valvular heart disease (e.g. worsening AS or MR)
- Progression of myocardial disease (e.g. dilated cardiomyopathy)
- Drugs (e.g. β-blockers or other negative inotropes or negative chronotropes)
- Infection (e.g. pneumonia, urinary tract infection, cellulitis, endocarditis)
- Non-cardiac medical conditions (e.g. anaemia, thyroid dysfunction, infection)
- Pulmonary disease (e.g. pulmonary hypertension [PHT] or pulmonary embolism [PE]).

There are many causes of *acute* heart failure (Box 4.1), the most common of which is myocardial infarction or ischaemia.

4.2 ASSESSMENT OF LV SYSTOLIC FUNCTION

This is one of the most important and common uses of echo. LV systolic function is a major prognostic factor in cardiac disease and has important implications for treatment. Clinical management is altered if an abnormality is detected (e.g. the diagnosis of systolic heart failure should lead to the initiation of ACE inhibitors unless there is a contraindication).

LV systolic function can be assessed by M-mode, 2-D and Doppler techniques. M-mode gives excellent resolution and allows measurement of LV dimensions and wall thickness. 2-D techniques are often used to provide a visual assessment of LV systolic function, both regional and global. The general validity of this has been shown but there are inter-observer variations. Visual estimation is clinically useful but unreliable in those who have poor echo images, can be limited in value in serial evaluation and inadequate where LV volumes critically influence the timing of intervention. Computer software on the echo machine may provide a quantitative assessment of LV function. Certain geometrical assumptions are made about LV shape that are not always valid, particularly in diseased hearts.

M-mode can be used to assess LV cavity dimensions, wall motion and thickness (Fig. 4.1). The phrase, 'a big heart is a bad heart', carries an important element of truth – poor LV systolic function is usually associated with increased LV dimensions. This is not always the case,

Box 4.1 Causes of acute heart failure and cardiogenic shock

• Acute MI – extensive LV myocardial damage, acute VSD, acute MR, RV infarction, cardiac rupture
• Decompensation of chronic heart failure – poor compliance with medication, intercurrent illness or infection, arrhythmia (e.g. AF or VT), myocardial ischaemia, anaemia, thyroid disease
• Arrhythmia – tachycardia (e.g. AF, VT or SVT) or bradycardia (e.g. complete heart block)
• Obstruction to cardiac output – critical aortic or mitral stenosis, HOCM, myxoma
• Valvular regurgitation – acute mitral or aortic regurgitation
• Myocarditis
• Acute massive pulmonary embolism
• Myocardial dysfunction following cardiac surgery
• Fluid overload
• Cardiac tamponade
• Cor pulmonale
• Poisoning or drug overdose
• Accelerated hypertension
• Cardiac trauma
• Rejection of heart transplant
• 'High output' heart failure (see Table 4.1).

Adapted from Holmberg S. Acute heart failure. In: Julian DG, Camm AJ, Fox KM et al, eds. Diseases of the Heart, 2nd ed. London: Saunders; 1996:456–466 and Dobb GJ. Cardiogenic shock. In: Oh TE, ed. Oh's Intensive Care Manual, 4th ed. Oxford: Butterworth-Heinemann; 1997:146-152.

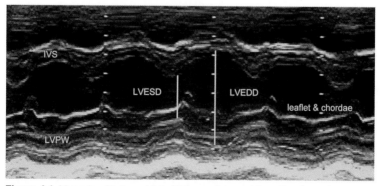

Figure 4.1 M-mode of left ventricle. This can be used to estimate cavity dimensions in systole and diastole, and wall thickness. It is important to identify the continuous endocardial echo and to distinguish this from echoes from chordae or mitral valve leaflet tips.

for example, if there is a large akinetic segment of LV wall or an apical LV aneurysm following MI, systolic function may be impaired due to regional wall motion abnormalities but M-mode measurements of LV dimensions may be within the normal range.

LV internal dimension measurements in end-systole (LVESD) and end-diastole (LVEDD) are made at the level of the MV leaflet tips in the parasternal long-axis view. Measurements are taken from the endocardium of the left surface of the interventricular septum (IVS) to the endocardium of the LV posterior wall (LVPW). The ultrasound beam should be as perpendicular as possible to the IVS. Care must be taken to distinguish between the endocardial surfaces and the chordae tendineae on the M-mode tracing.

LVEDD is at the end of diastole (R wave of ECG). The normal range is 3.8–5.8 cm.

LVESD is at the end of systole, which occurs at the peak downward motion of the IVS (which usually slightly precedes the peak upward motion of the LVPW) and coincides with the T wave on the ECG. The normal range is 2.2–4.0 cm.

Remember that the normal range for LVEDD and LVESD varies with several factors, including height, sex and age.

M-mode measurements can be converted to estimates of volume but this is inaccurate in regional LV dysfunction and spherical ventricles. The LVEDD and LVESD measurements can be used to calculate LV fractional shortening (FS), LV ejection fraction (EF) and LV volume, which give some further indication of LV systolic function.

Fractional shortening (FS) is a commonly used measure and is the percentage change in LV internal dimensions (not volumes) between systole and diastole:

$$FS = \frac{LVEDD - LVESD}{LVEDD} \times 100\%$$

Normal range is 25–45%.

The LV volume is derived from the 'cubed equation' (i.e. volume, $V = D^3$, where D is the ventricular dimension measured by M-mode). This assumes that the LV cavity is an ellipse shape, which is not always correct. There are some equations that attempt to improve the accuracy of this technique. The volume in end-diastole is estimated as $(LVEDD)^3$ and in end-systole as $(LVESD)^3$. The **ejection fraction (EF)** is the percentage change in LV volume between systole and diastole and is:

$$EF = \frac{(LVEDD)^3 - (LVESD)^3}{(LVEDD)^3} \times 100\%$$

The **normal ranges** for LV EF are shown below, as are EF ranges associated with different degrees of abnormality of LV systolic function.

LV ejection fraction – normal ranges and EF ranges with degree of abnormality of LV systolic function

	Normal	Mildly abnormal	Moderately abnormal	Severely abnormal
Women	54–74%	41–53%	30–40%	<30%
Men	52–72%	41–51%	30–40%	<30%

Based upon Lang et al. J Am Soc Echocardiogr. *2015;28:1-39.*

LV wall motion and changes in thickness during systole can be measured. The IVS moves towards the LVPW and the amplitude of this motion can be used as an indicator of LV function.

Wall thickness can also be measured. The walls thicken during systole. The normal range of thickness at end-diastole is 6–10 mm. Walls thinner than 6 mm may be stretched as in dilated cardiomyopathy or scarred and damaged by previous MI. Walls of thickness over 12 mm may indicate LV hypertrophy, an important independent prognostic factor in cardiovascular outcome risk.

2-D echo can be used qualitatively to assess LV systolic function by viewing the LV in a number of different planes and views. An experienced echo operator can often give a reasonably good visual assessment of LV systolic function as being normal, or mildly, moderately or severely impaired, and whether abnormalities are global or regional.

2-D echo can also be used to estimate LV volumes and EF. Multiple algorithms may be used to estimate LV volumes from 2-D images but all make some geometrical assumptions that may be invalid. The area–length method (symmetrical ventricles) and the apical bi-plane summation of discs method (asymmetrical ventricles) are validated and normal values are available.

Several techniques are available. **Simpson's method** (Fig. 4.2) divides the LV cavity into multiple slices of known thickness and diameter D (by taking multiple short-axis views at different levels along the LV long-axis) and then calculating the volume of each slice (area × thickness). The area is $\pi(D/2)^2$. The thinner the slices, the more accurate the estimate of LV volume. Calculations can be made by the computer of most echo machines. The endocardial border must be traced accurately and this is often the major technical difficulty. Endocardial definition has improved with some newer echo technology (e.g. harmonic imaging) and automated endocardial border detection systems are available on some echo machines. The computer calculates LV volume by dividing the apical view into 20 sections along the LV long-axis.

The LVEF can be obtained from LV volumes in systole and diastole (as above). Alternatively, computer-derived data can be obtained by taking and tracing the LV endocardial borders of a systolic and a diastolic LV frame.

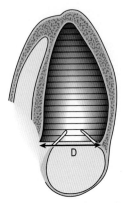

Figure 4.2 Simpson's method to estimate left ventricular volume.

An estimate of cardiac output can be obtained using LV volumes:

Cardiac output = stroke volume × heart rate

Stroke volume = LV diastolic volume – LV systolic volume.

Measurements of LV shape are an important and underutilized aspect of LV remodelling (e.g. after MI). Increasing LV sphericity has prognostic importance and loss of the normal LV shape may be an early indicator of LV dysfunction. 2-D echo allows a simple assessment of LV shape (measuring the ratio of long-axis length to mid-cavity diameter).

The location and extent of wall motion abnormality following MI correlate with LVEF and are prognostically useful.

Assessment of LV systolic function has been enhanced by newer echo techniques, such as 3-D echo (Section 5.4).

REGIONAL LV WALL MOTION

The LV can be divided up on 2-D imaging of apical 4-chamber and parasternal short-axis views into segments (16 or 17) and an assessment can be made of these segments (see Figs. 5.13, 5.14). This can be useful at rest and in stress echo to determine the location of coronary artery disease (Section 5.2).

A segment's systolic movement may be classified as:

• Normal
• Hypokinetic (reduced movement)
• Akinetic (no movement)
• Dyskinetic (movement in the wrong direction, e.g. outwards movement of the LV free wall during LV systole)
• Aneurysmal (out-pouching of all layers of the wall).

USEFUL INFORMATION FROM ECHO IN PATIENTS WITH HEART FAILURE

Left ventricle

- Dimensions – systolic and diastolic
- Systolic function and an indication of fractional shortening and ejection fraction
- Regional or global wall motion abnormalities – evidence of previous infarction, ischaemia or aneurysm
- Wall thickness – concentric hypertrophy (e.g. hypertension or amyloid) or asymmetrical hypertrophy (e.g. HCM)
- Evidence of diastolic heart failure.

Valves

- Aortic stenosis or regurgitation
- Mitral regurgitation – as a cause of heart failure or secondary to ventricular dilatation ('functional')
- Mitral stenosis.

Pericardium

- Effusion
- Constriction
- Echo suggestion of cardiac tamponade (e.g. RV diastolic collapse).

Right heart

- Right ventricular dimensions
- PHT (estimation of PASP by Doppler assessment of TR).

Left atrium

- Dimensions (particularly if AF and planned cardioversion).

Intracardiac thrombus

Changes in heart size and function in response to therapy

4.3 CORONARY ARTERY DISEASE

Echo plays an increasingly important role in assessing coronary artery disease. Resting and stress echo (Chapter 5) techniques are used in:

- Assessment of extent of ischaemia or infarction
- Prediction of artery causing ischaemia
- MI – LV function acutely and post MI, ischaemic cardiomyopathy

- RV infarction
- Complications of MI – MR, VSD, mural thrombus, LV aneurysm, pseudoaneurysm, effusion, rupture
- Coronary artery abnormalities (e.g. aneurysm, anomalous origin by transthoracic echo and TOE)
- Chest pain with normal coronaries – AS, HCM, MV prolapse.

ASSESSMENT OF ISCHAEMIA

Ischaemia results in immediate changes which can be detected by echo:
- Abnormalities of wall motion (hypokinetic, akinetic, dyskinetic)*
- Abnormalities of wall thickening (reduced or absent systolic thickening or systolic thinning – this is more sensitive and specific for ischaemia)*
- Abnormalities of overall LV function (e.g. ejection fraction).

(* also known as asynergy).

These can be detected by 2-D echo but M-mode is also extremely good because its high sampling rate makes it very sensitive to wall motion and thickening abnormalities. It is essential that the beam is at 90° to the wall. There are limited regions of the LV myocardium that can be examined by M-mode – most usefully, the posterior wall and IVS (Fig. 4.3).

The changes reverse if ischaemia is reversed, e.g. by rest, anti-anginal medication, percutaneous transluminal coronary angioplasty, thrombolysis or coronary artery bypass grafting (CABG). If the myocardium has its blood supply occluded for more than 1 h, permanent changes occur that include MI and scarring.

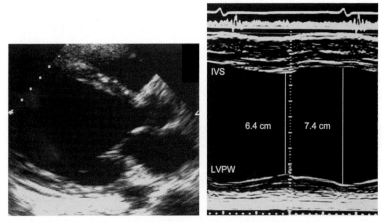

Figure 4.3 Dilated left ventricle with impaired systolic function due to coronary artery disease.

PREDICTION OF ARTERY INVOLVED

This is done by dividing the LV into segments as described (see Figs. 5.13 and 5.14). Stress echo is based on this.

ASSESSMENT OF MYOCARDIAL INFARCTION

Echo can help in detecting the extent of LV infarction, assessing RV involvement and detecting complications. The changes in LV function with acute MI are similar to those described for ischaemia, but rapidly become irreversible. Detection of RV involvement is important in determining treatment and prognosis (Section 4.6).

COMPLICATIONS OF MYOCARDIAL INFARCTION

Many of the complications of acute MI can be detected by echo.

- **Acute heart failure due to extensive MI.** This leads to pump failure, which may result in cardiogenic shock. Echo shows severe LV impairment.

In the following 2 complications (acute MR and acute VSD), LV systolic function is very active, unlike the situation above.

- **Acute MR.** This may be due to papillary muscle dysfunction or rupture (Fig. 4.4) or chordal rupture, which may be shown by 2-D echo. There may be a flail MV leaflet. The MR jet can be seen on continuous wave or colour flow mapping Doppler.

- **Acute VSD.** This is often near the cardiac apex and is more common in inferior and RV infarction. A discontinuity in the IVS can be seen on 2-D echo in the apical 4-chamber, parasternal long-axis and short-axis views. Colour flow mapping can show the defect. Pulsed wave Doppler moved along the RV side of the IVS

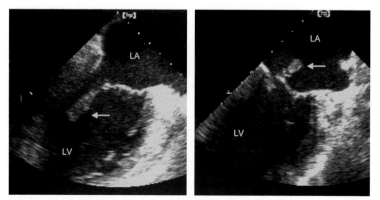

Figure 4.4 Papillary muscle rupture following acute myocardial infarction. The muscle (arrows) and the posterior mitral valve leaflet can be seen to prolapse into the left atrium. TOE study.

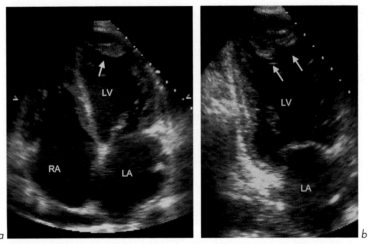

Figure 4.5 Thrombus in the apex of the left ventricle (arrows) following myocardial infarction. **(a)** Apical 4-chamber view and **(b)** apical 2-chamber view showing 2 distinct masses.

(parasternal long-axis or sometimes 4-chamber views) can show the jet.

- **Mural thrombus** (Fig. 4.5). This is shown on 2-D echo. It is usually located near an infarcted segment or aneurysm.

- **LV aneurysm.** Most frequently seen at or near the apex. More common in anterior than inferior MI. Best seen on 2-D echo. These can vary in size from small to very large, sometimes larger than the LV.

- **Pseudoaneurysm (false aneurysm).** This is rare. It follows rupture of the LV free wall and leads to haemopericardium (blood in the pericardial space), tamponade and is usually rapidly fatal. Sometimes, the haemopericardium clots and seals off the hole in the LV and a pseudoaneurysm forms. 2-D echo is a good way to diagnose this. It is important to detect, as it needs urgent surgical resection before it ruptures. It can be difficult to distinguish it from a true aneurysm but the communicating neck is usually narrower than the diameter of the aneurysm, the walls are thinner and its size changes in the cardiac cycle (expands in systole) and it is more often filled with thrombus.

- **Pericardial effusion** complicating MI can be detected by M-mode or 2-D echo.

- **Myocardial function after MI.** This gives an indication of prognosis. The scarred myocardium is seen as a thin segment that does not thicken during systole and has abnormal motion. Echo can assess the extent of MI, evaluate LV systolic and diastolic function, and look at residual complications.

MYOCARDIAL 'HIBERNATION' AND 'STUNNING'

The heart is critically dependent upon its blood supply. Occlusion of a coronary artery results in the cessation of myocardial contraction within 1 min. Myocardial cell death usually occurs after 15 min of ischaemia.

An impairment of contractile function may remain even after restoration of the blood supply without MI. This effect has been termed *myocardial stunning* (stunned heart). It may cause reversible systolic or diastolic dysfunction. Although stunned myocardium is viable, normal function may not be regained for up to 2 weeks. Recurrent episodes of ischaemia may result in the loss of normal function of the heart, and the term *hibernating myocardium* (hibernation) has been applied to a similar condition.

ECHO ASSESSMENT OF CORONARY ARTERY ANATOMY

Echo is not yet able to give a very accurate assessment of most parts of the coronary anatomy. The origins of the left and right coronary arteries may be seen in some transthoracic echo studies by using a modified parasternal short-axis view at the AV level.

Abnormalities are more likely to be seen during TOE, e.g.
- Anomalous origin of coronaries (e.g. origin from PA)
- Coronary artery fistula (Fig. 4.6)

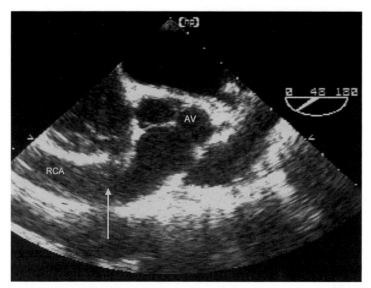

Figure 4.6 Huge dilatation of the right coronary artery (RCA, arrow) due to coronary fistula. TOE short-axis study at aortic valve level.

- Aneurysm (e.g. Kawasaki syndrome, an acquired condition in children with coronary aneurysms that may be several centimetres in diameter).

4.4 CARDIOMYOPATHIES AND MYOCARDITIS

The cardiomyopathies are a diverse group of disorders. Cardiomyopathy means heart muscle abnormality, and strictly speaking the term should be applied to conditions that have no known underlying cause. These are known as idiopathic cardiomyopathies. The term has been extended to include conditions where there is an underlying cause (e.g. alcoholic, ischaemic, hypertensive cardiomyopathy, etc.)

The most important idiopathic cardiomyopathies are:
- Hypertrophic (increased ventricular wall thickness)
- Dilated (increased ventricular volume)
- Restrictive (increased ventricular stiffness).

1. HYPERTROPHIC CARDIOMYOPATHY

This is an autosomal dominant condition with a high mutation rate (up to 50% of cases are sporadic). It is rare with an incidence of 0.4–2.5 per 100 000 per year. A number of mutations of cardiac proteins have been identified as underlying causes. These include β-myosin heavy chain, myosin-binding protein C, α-tropomyosin and troponin T (TnT).

The clinical features include:
- Angina with normal coronary arteries – due to ventricular hypertrophy and myocardial oxygen supply/demand imbalance
- Arrhythmias
- Breathlessness
- Syncope
- Sudden cardiac death (SCD; annual death rate is 3% in adults) – due to outflow tract obstruction or arrhythmia
- Ejection systolic murmur, which may be confused with valvular aortic stenosis
- Heart failure (10–15%).

The characteristic feature is myocardial hypertrophy in any part of the ventricular wall:
- IVS to a greater extent than the free wall (termed asymmetrical septal hypertrophy or ASH) – 60% of cases
- Concentric – 30% of cases
- Apical – 10% of cases
- RV hypertrophy – 30% of cases and correlates with severity of LVH.

Hypertrophy, particularly of the septum, may cause left ventricular outflow tract obstruction (LVOTO). In this situation, the term hypertrophic *obstructive* cardiomyopathy (HOCM) is appropriate. This 'dynamic' obstruction becomes more pronounced in the later stages of systole. As the LV empties, the LV cavity size becomes smaller and the anterior MV leaflet moves anteriorly to contact the septum. It may be present at rest or become more pronounced with exercise. In some people with HCM, the most dangerous time is at the end of vigorous exercise, e.g. at half-time in a football match. At this time, ventricular volumes diminish as cardiac output and heart rate decrease, catecholamine drive decreases and there may be changes in circulating electrolyte concentrations, such as potassium ions (K^+). These features all combine to increase the risk of syncope and sudden death by increasing the likelihood of LVOTO and arrhythmias.

Echo is diagnostic of HCM. The important echo features are seen using both **M-mode** and **2-D imaging**:

1. ASH (Fig. 4.7)
2. Systolic anterior motion (SAM) of the MV apparatus, which may abut the IVS. This may not be seen at rest but may occur following provocation by the Valsalva manoeuvre or isovolumic exercise
3. Mid-systolic AV closure and fluttering.

The definition of asymmetrical hypertrophy varies but a septal to posterior wall ratio of 1.5 or more is unequivocal evidence of asymmetry.

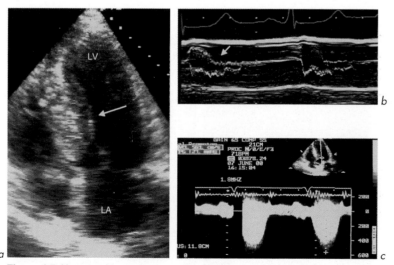

Figure 4.7 Hypertrophic cardiomyopathy. **(a)** Asymmetrical septal hypertrophy (arrow). **(b)** Fluttering and premature mid-systolic closure of the aortic valve (arrow). **(c)** Continuous Doppler showing a peak velocity across the left ventricular outflow tract of 5.6 m/s (estimated peak gradient 127 mmHg).

Neither ASH nor SAM is specific for HCM. ASH may occur in AS and SAM may occur in MV prolapse. Their occurrence together is strongly suggestive of HCM.

Continuous wave Doppler shows increased peak flow through the LVOT. Pulsed wave Doppler with the sample volume in the LVOT proximal to the AV shows that the increase in velocity occurs below the level of the valve, distinguishing the obstruction from valvular AS. The peak in maximal velocity across the AV is often bifid in HCM. There may also be features of LV diastolic dysfunction due to LVH (e.g. abnormal transmitral flow pattern with E-wave smaller than A-wave, Section 4.5).

Treatment of HCM is based on the person's symptoms and physical signs, family history and risk factors. Options include medications (e.g. β-blockers), consideration for implantable cardioverter-defibrillator (ICD) and/or reduction of LVOTO by septal reduction, either by surgical myomectomy (LV muscle excision) or by catheter techniques to instil ethanol to cause septal ablation (see Fig. 5.15).

2. DILATED CARDIOMYOPATHY

This is characterized by dilatation of the cardiac chambers, particularly the LV (although all other chambers are often involved) with reduced wall thickness and reduced wall motion (Fig. 4.8). The incidence is estimated at 6.0 per 100 000 per year. Most cases are isolated although some familial forms have been identified. The reduced LV wall motion is usually global rather than regional, as seen in LV systolic impairment due to coronary artery disease (ischaemia or infarction).

M-mode and **2-D echo** show:
- Dilatation of all the cardiac chambers (left and right ventricles and atria) – increased LVESD and LVEDD

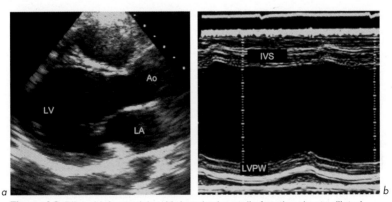

Figure 4.8 Dilated left ventricle with impaired systolic function due to dilated cardiomyopathy. **(a)** Parasternal long-axis view and **(b)** M-mode.

- Reduced wall thickness and motion (ranging from mild to severe impairment) – reduced ejection fraction and fractional shortening, reduced motion of IVS and LVPW
- Intracardiac thrombus (LV and LA).

Doppler studies may show functional MR and TR.

Several conditions give rise to a clinical picture that is similar to idiopathic dilated cardiomyopathy. These include toxins such as alcohol and certain drugs, especially those used in the treatment of some cancers.

Cancer chemotherapy

Chemotherapy with doxorubicin produces a dose-dependent degenerative cardiomyopathy. Other cancer drugs (e.g. trastuzumab) may cause LV dysfunction and/or heart failure. Baseline and re-evaluation echo should be carried out in individuals receiving cancer drugs. Cumulative doses of doxazosin should usually be kept to below 400 mg/m^2. Subtle abnormalities of LV systolic function (increased wall stress) are found in approximately 1 in 6 patients receiving only one dose of doxorubicin. Most patients who receive at least 228 mg/m^2 show either reduced contractility or increased wall stress. Early abnormalities of diastolic function (in the absence of systolic abnormalities) may occur in patients receiving 200–300 mg/m^2.

A detailed description of the role of echo in individuals with cancer is given in Section 7.9.

3. RESTRICTIVE CARDIOMYOPATHY

This is characterized by increased myocardial stiffness or impaired relaxation and abnormal diastolic function of one or both ventricles. Several disorders give rise to a clinical picture of restrictive cardiomyopathy:
1. Idiopathic
2. Infiltrations – amyloid, sarcoid, haemochromatosis, glycogen storage diseases (e.g. Pompe's), mucopolysaccharidoses (e.g. Gaucher's, Fabry's)
3. Endomyocardial fibrosis – hypereosinophilic syndrome (Loeffler's endomyocardial fibrosis), carcinoid, malignancy.

The echo assessment is difficult and the features are not specific. If features of restrictive cardiomyopathy are present, evidence of myocardial infiltration or endomyocardial fibrosis should be sought. The echo differentiation between restrictive cardiomyopathy and constrictive pericarditis can be difficult but is important as it has management implications (Section 4.8).

Echo features of restrictive cardiomyopathy

- LV and RV cavity sizes are usually normal or only mildly increased, but there is impaired contractility of the ventricular walls seen on M-mode and 2-D echo. There may be dilatation of the LA and RA.
- Impaired LV and RV diastolic function. This is best assessed by Doppler echo. There is often a characteristic abnormal 'restrictive pattern' of MV flow with a very large E-wave and small A-wave (Section 4.5).

Infiltration

The findings are similar whatever the underlying cause. Amyloid is the most common infiltrative disease (Fig. 4.9). The features are:
- Concentric thickening of the LV and RV free walls and septum and the interatrial septum
- LV and RV internal dimensions are often reduced
- Reduced wall and septal motion
- Failure of systolic thickening of the IVS and LV free wall
- Patches of high-intensity 'speckling' in the hypertrophied muscle
- Thickening of the MV and TV leaflets with regurgitation (aortic and pulmonary valves may also be thickened)
- Pericardial effusion
- LV diastolic impairment with or without systolic impairment
- Intracardiac thrombus.

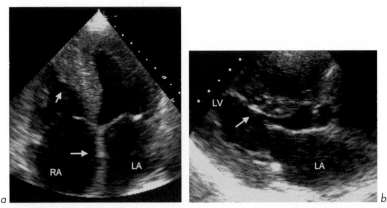

Figure 4.9 Amyloid heart disease. **(a)** Left ventricular and right ventricular hypertrophy, with apical obliteration of the right ventricular cavity with thrombus (arrow). The atria are dilated and the interatrial septum is thickened (arrow), as are the valve leaflets. **(b)** Hypertrophy and speckling of the interventricular septum (arrow).

Endomyocardial fibrosis

- Cavity obliteration especially at the RV and LV apex due to fibrosis or eosinophilic infiltration
- Bright echogenic endocardium
- Normal or thickened LV walls with reduced contractility
- Normal LV or reduced cavity size
- Similar changes in RV to LV
- Dilated RA and LA
- Intracardiac thrombus
- LV diastolic impairment with or without systolic impairment.

The echo features differentiating restrictive cardiomyopathy from constrictive pericarditis are discussed in Section 4.8.

4. OTHER CARDIOMYOPATHIES

Some cardiomyopathies have specific echo features. These include:
- LV non-compaction
- Takotsubo cardiomyopathy
- Arrhythmogenic cardiomyopathy (AC; also known as arrhythmogenic RV cardiomyopathy [ARVC] or dysplasia [ARVD]).

LV non-compaction ('spongy myocardium')

This is a rare condition with a reported prevalence between 0.014% and 1.3% in the population, based on echo studies.

There is a distinctive appearance on **2-D echo** (Fig. 4.10). There are areas of normal ('compact') and abnormal, spongy ('non-compact') myocardium, usually at the LV apex and lateral free wall. Some individuals have a meshwork of trabeculations or multiple prominent trabeculations. These have blood-filled recesses, which communicate with the LV cavity and can be seen on colour flow mapping. Note that LV trabeculations may be seen in some normal individuals. Apical HCM or thrombus may give similar appearances. Because echo visualization of the LV apex is poor in some cases, cardiac magnetic resonance imaging (MRI) can be used to confirm the diagnosis.

LV non-compaction usually presents in childhood or early adulthood. It is thought to be due to a developmental abnormality, probably caused by arrested compaction during intrauterine development. There may be an associated congenital cardiac abnormality. It may have an underlying genetic inheritance in at least 30–50% of cases. Several genes that lead to LV non-compaction have been identified. These generally encode sarcomeric (contractile apparatus) or cytoskeletal proteins. When LV non-compaction is associated with congenital heart disease, disturbance of the Notch signalling pathway seems part of the final common pathway. Some

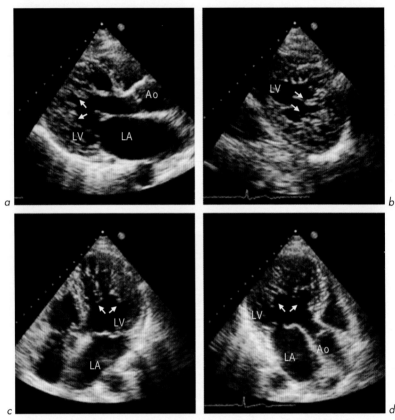

Figure 4.10 Left ventricular non-compaction. Prominent LV trabeculations (arrows). **(a)** Parasternal long-axis view. **(b)** Parasternal short-axis view. **(c)** Apical 4-chamber view. **(d)** Apical long-axis view. Images adapted from Souza O, Silva G, Sampaio F, et al. Isolated left ventricular non-compaction: a single-center experience. *Rev Port Cardiol.* 2013;32:229–238, with permission.

cases are caused by disturbed mitochondrial function or are due to metabolic abnormalities.

There is an increased risk of a triad of complications: heart failure, life-threatening ventricular arrhythmias and systemic thromboembolism.

There are some unresolved issues:

- True prevalence may be underestimated or overestimated in the population
- Further understanding of genetic basis
- Definitive echo and cardiac MRI diagnostic criteria are needed
- Prevalence and diagnosis of RV involvement
- Whether prognosis is changed by early diagnosis and treatment.

Takotsubo cardiomyopathy ('broken heart syndrome' or 'stress cardiomyopathy')

This was described by Satoh and co-workers in Japan in 1990. Takotsubo is a Japanese term meaning a fishing pot for catching octopuses (tako = octopus, tsubo = jar/pot/vase). The term is used because, in this condition, the LV is said to resemble this shape on end-systolic LV ventriculography (Fig. 4.11).

This cardiomyopathy is estimated to affect between 1.2% and 2.2% of people in Japan and between 2% and 3% in Western countries. It affects far more women (approximately 90% of cases) than men. Most cases occur after the menopause, with the usual age at onset between 58 and 75 years, mean age of 68 years and it is more prevalent in the 7th and 8th decades of life. Less than 3% of reported cases occurred in people under 50 years of age.

The presentation is usually with severe chest pain, suggestive of acute MI. The incidence is estimated as 0.7–2.5% of those initially presenting with an acute coronary syndrome. It may be triggered by intense emotional stress (hence 'broken heart'), physical stress, or by medical procedures or surgery. Over 85% of reported cases follow either a physically or emotionally stressful event. Examples include grief from the death of a loved one, fear from public speaking, arguing with a spouse, relationship disagreements or financial problems. Cases have been reported triggered by acute asthma, surgery, chemotherapy, stroke and near-drowning.

ECG changes occur and may include ST-segment elevation in the precordial leads, T-wave inversion, pathological Q-waves, QT prolongation or new bundle branch block (left [LBBB] or right bundle branch block [RBBB]). Blood biomarkers of cardiac damage (e.g. troponins, creatine phosphokinase) are usually elevated.

Crucially, coronary angiography does not demonstrate significant coronary artery obstruction or occlusion.

The pathophysiology is still unclear. Suggested mechanisms include:

- Multi-vessel spasm of epicardial coronary arteries
- Acute microvascular spasm
- Excessive sympathetic stimulation. Markedly elevated serum concentrations of catecholamines may induce myocardial metabolic impairment and stunning
- Neurogenic stunned myocardium caused by acute autonomic dysfunction
- Transient coronary occlusion with thrombus, with reperfusion due to spontaneous lysis.

Irrespective of its underlying aetiology, it has been hypothesized that takotsubo cardiomyopathy may be characterized by a common pathophysiological pattern involving acute and reversible coronary

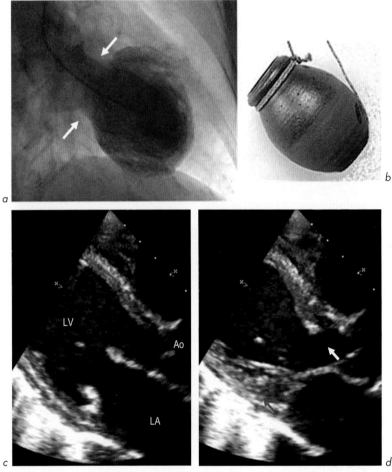

Figure 4.11 Takotsubo cardiomyopathy. **(a)** Contrast left ventriculogram showing a typical takotsubo LV shape at end-systole. There is a narrow neck (arrows) with apical ballooning (spherical shape) of the LV, similar to the shape of the **(b)** Takotsubo (pot for fishing octopuses). **(c)** Off-axis parasternal long-axis echo view in a patient with takotsubo cardiomyopathy showing dilated LV in end-diastole. **(d)** End-systolic view in the same patient, showing contraction of upper septum (anterior basal septal segment, white arrow – see Figure 5.13) and upper posterior wall (posterobasal segment, red arrow) but poor contraction of lower septum and posterior wall (anterior apical septal and diaphragmatic segments), giving a takotsubo appearance. Images (a) and (b) adapted from Cesário V, Loureiro MJ, Pereira H. Takotsubo cardiomyopathy in a cardiology department. *Rev Port Cardiol.* 2012;31:603–608, with permission.

microvascular dysfunction. The occurrence of the syndrome in post-menopausal women may support the hypothesis of stress-mediated vasoconstriction enhanced by oestrogen depletion. **Echo** is crucial in making the diagnosis. This typically shows ballooning of the LV apex with reduced LVEF, which may be severe. There may be an apical LV aneurysm with full-thickness myocardium. There is extensive akinesia of most of the LV (particularly LV apex, distal anterior wall and lateral segments) with compensatory hyperkinesis of basal LV segments. There may be SAM of the MV and MR.

Patients are usually very ill with severe heart failure, but subsequently recover. Complete recovery of LV function and of the LV aneurysm within a few days or weeks after admission is typical. Echo may also detect complications, which include apical LV thrombus and pericardial effusion. 2-D echo in the acute phase plays a crucial role in making the diagnosis and also with follow-up. 3-D echo is also useful. Other helpful techniques are nuclear myocardial perfusion imaging, computed tomography (CT) and cardiac MRI. Ventriculography at the time of cardiac catheterization demonstrates the takotsubo-shaped LV (Fig. 4.11). The LV is predominantly affected, but cases with LV and RV involvement have been described.

To make this clinical diagnosis, these diagnostic criteria have been suggested:

1. Acute onset with stressful trigger
2. New ECG abnormalities (as above)
3. Elevated cardiac biomarkers
4. Echo showing transient ballooning of LV with apical, distal anterior and lateral severe hypokinesia or akinesia, beyond a single coronary artery distribution (unlike most acute MI)
5. Non-obstructive coronary artery disease at angiography
6. Absence of: myocarditis, phaeochromocytoma, head trauma or intracranial haemorrhage, HCM
7. Recovery of LV function, usually within 12 weeks.

The treatment of takotsubo cardiomyopathy is generally supportive and needs to be individualized for each patient. Since there is a high catecholamine state, patients should not be given inotropes. Treatment may include intra-aortic balloon pump, fluids, and β-blockers or calcium channel blockers. Aspirin is usually commenced, but discontinued after acute MI has been excluded. Some reports suggest anticoagulation therapy. The role of vasodilators such as endothelin antagonists and adenosine may be considered in future trials. Treatment should include lifestyle changes. Individuals should stay physically healthy, whilst learning and maintaining methods to manage stress, to cope with future difficult situations.

Despite the initial presentation, most patients survive the acute event, with a very low rate of in-hospital mortality or complications. Long-term prognosis is excellent. Even when LV systolic function is heavily compromised at presentation, it typically improves within the first few days and normalizes within a few months. Infrequent recurrence has been reported and seems to be associated with the nature of the trigger.

Arrhythmogenic cardiomyopathy (AC) – also known as arrhythmogenic RV cardiomyopathy or dysplasia (ARVC, ARVD)

AC is a genetic cardiomyopathy that involves primarily the RV. LV involvement becomes present in a majority of cases and a left dominant form has also been described. It is thus best referred to as arrhythmogenic cardiomyopathy (AC) rather than ARVC or ARVD. It is characterized by fibrous fatty replacement of the myocardium, starting at the epicardium and extending transmurally. There are hypokinetic areas involving the RV free wall, with associated arrhythmias originating in the RV.

It usually shows an autosomal dominant pattern with variable penetrance (not all carriers of the gene show the clinical manifestations). Approximately 40–50% of AC patients have a mutation identified in one of several genes encoding desmosomal proteins (proteins that bind cells to one another) such as plakoglobin and desmoplakin.

AC is seen predominantly in males, and 30–50% of cases have a familial distribution. The incidence is reported as 1 in 1000 to 1 in 10000 in the population in the US. In some studies, 1 in 200 were found to be carriers of mutations that predispose to AC. It accounts for up to 17% of all cases of sudden cardiac death (SCD) in young people. The penetrance is 20–35% in general, but significantly higher in some countries, such as Italy. In Italy, the incidence is estimated at 40 in 10000, making it the most common cause of SCD in young people.

AC clinical presentations vary. Ventricular arrhythmias, syncope and SCD are the most severe. Up to 80% of people with AC present with syncope or SCD. The remainder frequently present with palpitations or other symptoms due to RV outflow tract (RVOT) tachycardia (a type of monomorphic VT). Symptoms are usually exercise-related. In populations where HCM is screened out prior to involvement in competitive athletics, it is a common cause of SCD. AC may cause heart failure.

The first clinical signs of AC are usually during adolescence, but it has been demonstrated in infants. AC is an important cause of ventricular arrhythmias in children and young adults. Early diagnosis appears crucial in preventing SCD. Mortality in patients with AC receiving an ICD is relatively low. Diagnosing AC can be difficult and is currently based on the presence of major and minor Task Force criteria, which include ECG, structural (cardiac imaging and histology), clinical and familial factors. Beyond a personal and family medical history, assessment includes ECG (90% of people with AC have some ECG abnormality), echo, 24-hour ECG Holter monitoring, stress testing and cardiac MRI. In uncertain diagnoses, endocardial voltage mapping may help detect the presence of myocardial scarring in early disease. Myocardial biopsy may be used diagnostically.

Echo may reveal an enlarged, hypokinetic RV with a paper-thin RV free wall. RV dilatation causes dilatation of the TV annulus, with subsequent TR. Paradoxical septal motion may also be present.

Genetic testing is important. Children of an AC patient have a 50% chance of inheriting the disease-causing mutation. Whenever a mutation is found, family-specific genetic testing can be used to identify relatives who are at risk for the disease. All first-degree family members of the affected person should be screened. Screening should begin during the teenage years.

The goal of management of AC is to decrease the incidence of SCD. This may include asymptomatic individuals, diagnosed during family screening. Some people with AC are considered at high risk for SCD:

• Young age
• Competitive sports activity
• Malignant familial history
• Extensive RV disease with decreased RVEF
• LV involvement
• Syncope
• Episodes of ventricular arrhythmia.

Management options are pharmacological (antiarrhythmic drugs including β-blockers, such as sotalol, or amiodarone and anticoagulants to reduce thrombus formation and PE in people with decreased RVEF or with dyskinetic portions of the RV), radiofrequency catheter ablation, placement of an ICD or surgery. Cardiac transplantation may be indicated for uncontrollable arrhythmias or severe, uncontrollable heart failure.

Sporting activity is associated with increased risk of SCD in patients with AC. In addition, the overload resulting from training may accelerate progression. As AC is a disease of desmosomal dysfunction, factors increasing myocardial strain worsen the mechanical coupling between cardiac myocytes and promote myocardial replacement and fibrosis. When placed under mechanical

Table 4.2 Clinical management and prevention of sudden cardiac death (SCD) in patients with arrhythmogenic cardiomyopathy (AC)

Recommendations for all patients:
• Reduce physical exercise
• Avoid competitive sport
• Annual follow-up, including:
  – ECG
  – Cardiac imaging (echo or cardiac MRI)
  – Holter
  – Exercise stress testing

Additional recommendations for groups:

Group	Risk markers	Medication	ICD
Definite AC High risk	Aborted SCD Sustained VT Unexplained syncope	β-Blockers	Recommended
Definite AC Moderate risk	Extensive disease (severe RV dysfunction, large LV involvement) Non-sustained VT	β-Blockers	Consider
Definite AC Low risk	Remaining patients with definite diagnosis of AC	β-Blockers	Not recommended
Asymptomatic mutation carriers	Asymptomatic mutation-carrying relatives of AC	Not routinely	Not recommended

Adapted from Brugada J, Fernández-Armenta J. ESC E-Journal of Cardiology Practice at: <http://www.escardio.org/Guidelines-&-Education/Journals-and -publications/ESC-journals-family/E-journal-of-Cardiology-Practice/Volume-10/ Arrhythmogenic-right-ventricular-dyplasia>; 2012.

stress (exercise) the defective desmosomes may detach from each other, leading to cell death. This causes inflammation with scar formation and fat deposition. Therefore, patients with AC – including asymptomatic mutation carriers – should avoid strenuous physical exercise (Table 4.2). Competitive sports are altogether contraindicated and recommendations on recreational sport are very restrictive.

5. MYOCARDITIS

This is inflammation of the heart muscle. The underlying cause is often not found, but it may be due to:

- Viruses such as Coxsackie B, influenza
- Bacteria such as *Mycoplasma pneumoniae*
- Parasites, e.g. Chagas' disease, Lyme disease (Section 7.8)
- Toxins, e.g. ethanol, drugs, chemicals
- Connective tissue disease, e.g. SLE
- Fungi.

This is a clinical diagnosis and there may be a history suggestive of an underlying cause. ECG often shows a resting tachycardia with widespread T-wave inversion. The echo features are not specific and are similar to those of dilated cardiomyopathy, with impaired systolic and diastolic function and evidence of new valvular regurgitation (e.g. MR). Serial echo examinations may show a change in LV function or valvular abnormalities that would support the diagnosis of myocarditis rather than dilated cardiomyopathy. There may be regional LV wall motion abnormalities in myocarditis.

4.5 DIASTOLIC FUNCTION

Clinical features of left heart failure may occur in people with normal or near-normal LV systolic function assessed by echo, due to diastolic dysfunction, systolic impairment on exertion or ischaemia.

Diastolic function of the LV relates to chamber stiffness and relaxation following ventricular contraction. It is not a passive phenomenon and requires energy. Abnormalities of LV diastolic function occur in several conditions and can be assessed by echo but their assessment is rather complex. These abnormalities may co-exist with abnormalities of systolic function, or may occur in isolation or before systolic impairment becomes obvious.

Diastole has 4 phases (Fig. 4.12):

1. Isovolumic relaxation
2. Early rapid filling
3. Late filling
4. Atrial systole.

Abnormalities in any of these phases may contribute to diastolic heart failure.

Heart failure may be predominantly diastolic in one-third of cases. In these cases, echo measures of diastolic function can be abnormal. It is wise to assess LV systolic and diastolic function separately since the causes of abnormalities and, more importantly, their treatments, differ.

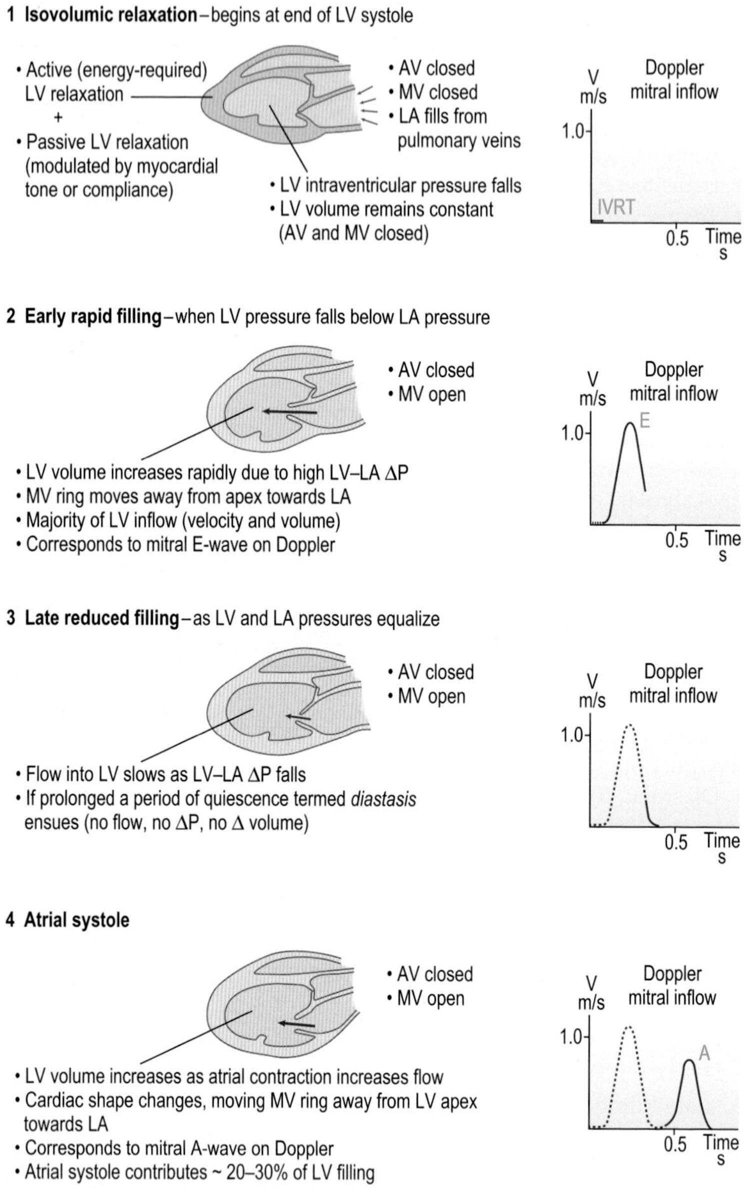

1 Isovolumic relaxation – begins at end of LV systole

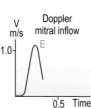

- Active (energy-required) LV relaxation
  +
- Passive LV relaxation (modulated by myocardial tone or compliance)

- AV closed
- MV closed
- LA fills from pulmonary veins

- LV intraventricular pressure falls
- LV volume remains constant (AV and MV closed)

Doppler mitral inflow

V m/s

1.0

IVRT

0.5 Time s

2 Early rapid filling – when LV pressure falls below LA pressure

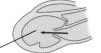

- AV closed
- MV open

- LV volume increases rapidly due to high LV–LA ΔP
- MV ring moves away from apex towards LA
- Majority of LV inflow (velocity and volume)
- Corresponds to mitral E-wave on Doppler

Doppler mitral inflow

V m/s

1.0

E

0.5 Time s

3 Late reduced filling – as LV and LA pressures equalize

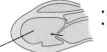

- AV closed
- MV open

- Flow into LV slows as LV–LA ΔP falls
- If prolonged a period of quiescence termed *diastasis* ensues (no flow, no ΔP, no Δ volume)

Doppler mitral inflow

V m/s

1.0

0.5 Time s

4 Atrial systole

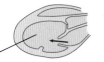

- AV closed
- MV open

- LV volume increases as atrial contraction increases flow
- Cardiac shape changes, moving MV ring away from LV apex towards LA
- Corresponds to mitral A-wave on Doppler
- Atrial systole contributes ~ 20–30% of LV filling

Doppler mitral inflow

V m/s

1.0

A

0.5 Time s

Figure 4.12 Phases of left ventricular diastole. A similar process occurs in the right ventricle.

Diastolic heart failure is common in elderly people and should be suspected in patients with symptoms of heart failure with normal size hearts and ventricular hypertrophy and/or myocardial ischaemia. Diastolic heart failure occurs in up to 50% of patients with heart failure in the community but is less common (<10%) in people admitted to hospital with heart failure.

LV diastolic dysfunction can be graded into: grade I (mild), grade II (moderate) and grade III (severe). This is described in detail below. Grading appears to be of prognostic significance.

CAUSES OF LV DIASTOLIC IMPAIRMENT

These often co-exist (e.g. hypertension and coronary artery disease):

1. Ageing effects
2. LV hypertrophy – hypertension, AS, HCM
3. Ischaemic heart disease
4. Restrictive cardiomyopathy
5. LV infiltrations – amyloid, sarcoid, carcinoid, haemochromatosis
6. Pericardial constriction.

In general, these are conditions that increase stiffness of the LV wall. LV relaxation is then abnormal, impairing diastolic flow from the LA into the LV. Diastolic function is more sensitive than systolic function to the effects of age and is very dependent on filling conditions.

Remember that from Newton's second law of motion (force = mass × acceleration), the only factor that causes blood to move from the LA to the LV is atrioventricular force (or pressure gradient, in mmHg/cm). Ventricular disease modifies diastolic LV filling by modifying this gradient. Blood acceleration, not blood velocity, is proportional to the atrioventricular pressure gradient. Peak blood velocity thus depends not only on the peak pressure gradient but also on the time during which it has acted.

ECHO ASSESSMENT OF LV DIASTOLIC FUNCTION

LV diastolic function is complex and dependent upon a number of factors such as age, preload, afterload, heart rate and the co-existence of other abnormalities (e.g. MV disease).

There is no good single echo measure. Doppler measurements of LV filling pattern should not necessarily be viewed as the only reflection of LV 'diastolic function'. It is a mistake to rely on single measurements such as E : A ratios (see below) and many anatomical and haemodynamic features should be considered together.

Surgically correctable conditions which mimic diastolic dysfunction such as constrictive pericarditis must be excluded by echo and, if necessary, other techniques such as MRI, CT scanning and cardiac catheterization.

Using **M-mode**, motion of the anterior mitral valve leaflet (AMVL) during diastole has a characteristic M-shaped (E–A) pattern, assuming that the person is in sinus rhythm and there is no MS. If the LV is stiffer than usual, abnormalities of AMVL motion may be observed, for example:

- Diminished AMVL excursion (E-wave)
- Increase in A-wave size (as atrial contraction contributes to a greater extent to diastolic filling of the LV)
- Reduced E : A ratio.

These are *not* specific or highly sensitive for LV diastolic impairment.

The normal LV myocardium relaxes without any increase in LV volume during the interval between closure of the AV (A_2) and opening of the MV. This is called the isovolumic relaxation time (IVRT) and is usually 50–80 ms. The IVRT often increases with diastolic dysfunction, but also normally increases with age (see below).

2-D echo does not help to make a direct assessment of LV diastolic dysfunction but can detect associated abnormalities such as:

- LV hypertrophy
- Myocardial infiltration (e.g. amyloid)
- Pericardial effusion and/or thickening
- Ischaemic heart disease (regional LV wall motion and thickening abnormalities or scarring)
- Dilated IVC
- **There may also be co-existent LV systolic abnormalities.**

Doppler can provide useful information regarding LV diastolic dysfunction but relying on measures of transmitral flow alone is not sufficient.

IVRT often increases with diastolic dysfunction, but also increases with age and changes with heart rate. Impaired relaxation is thus associated with a prolonged IVRT, whilst decreased compliance and elevated filling pressures are associated with a shortened IVRT. Thus, IVRT measurement is useful in determining the severity of diastolic dysfunction, particularly in serial studies of patients to assess response to medical therapy or disease progression. IVRT is measured from an apical 4-chamber view angulated anteriorly to show the LVOT and AV. Using pulsed wave Doppler, a 3–5 mm sample volume is positioned midway between the AV and MV to obtain a signal showing both aortic outflow and mitral inflow, ideally with a defined AV closing click. IVRT is measured as the time from the middle of the aortic closure click to the onset of mitral flow.

Mitral valve flow pattern and diastolic function

The MV diastolic flow pattern reflects flow into the LV. This can be assessed by pulsed Doppler using the apical 4-chamber view with the sample volume in the mitral orifice. Mitral flow pattern is influenced by a large number of factors. These include LV stiffness, preload, afterload, cardiac rhythm, conduction abnormalities, LA systolic function, heart rate, AR, MR and the phase of respiration.

In the normal heart, there is a characteristic flow pattern:
- The E-wave is the result of passive early diastolic LV filling
- The A-wave represents active late diastolic LV filling due to LA contraction
- The acceleration time (AT) and deceleration time (DT) of the E-wave can be measured. AT is the time from onset of diastolic flow to the peak of the E-wave. DT is the time from the E-wave peak to the point where the deceleration slope hits the baseline.

The E-wave is often greater than the A-wave but it is important to remember that this **varies with age**. The E-wave, E : A ratio and E-wave deceleration times tend to fall with increasing age.

Age- and gender-specific normal ranges for mitral flow-derived indices of LV diastolic function in a general population have been published. Approximate values are given in Tables 4.3A and 4.3B.

Three abnormal mitral flow patterns (reflecting LV filling) are recognized (Figs. 4.13, 4.14):

1. **'Impaired-relaxation (slow relaxation) pattern'.** Decreased LV relaxation due to mild diastolic dysfunction (grade I) associated with LV hypertrophy or myocardial ischaemia:
   - E-wave is small, A-wave is large, E : A ratio <1, AT prolonged, IVRT prolonged.

2. **'Pseudonormal pattern'.** More severe diastolic dysfunction (grade II) leads to increased LA pressure, which improves early passive filling, giving a mitral flow pattern that appears normal (distinguish from normal by presence of other abnormalities, e.g. LVH or LA enlargement):
   - E-wave velocity predominates, E : A ratio >1.

3. **'Restrictive pattern'.** Seen in severe diastolic dysfunction (grade III). Reduced LV filling may also be caused by restrictive cardiomyopathy or constrictive pericarditis (conditions causing a rapid rise of LV diastolic pressure). It may, however, occur in other conditions, such as with high LV filling pressures, systolic heart failure, MR and HCM:
   - E-wave very tall, A-wave is small, E ≫ A, DT short, IVRT short.

Table 4.3A Mitral flow indices

Sex differences in a large population study*	Men	Women
Peak E-wave (m/s)	0.66 ± 0.15	0.70 ± 0.16
E-wave deceleration time (s)	0.21 ± 0.04	0.20 ± 0.04
Peak A-wave (m/s)	0.67 ± 0.16	0.72 ± 0.18
E : A ratio	1.04 ± 0.38	1.03 ± 0.34

Data from Tromsø Study. Schirmer H, Lunde P, Rasmussen K. Mitral flow derived Doppler indices of left ventricular diastolic function in a general population: the Tromsø study. Eur Heart J. 2000;21:1376–1386.

Table 4.3B Mitral flow indices

Effects of age*	Age <50 years	Age >50 years
Peak E-wave (m/s)	0.72 ± 0.14	0.62 ± 0.14
E-wave deceleration time (s)	0.18 ± 0.02	0.21 ± 0.04
Peak A-wave (m/s)	0.40 ± 0.10	0.59 ± 0.14
E : A ratio	1.9 ± 0.6	1.1 ± 0.3

Data from Tromsø Study. Schirmer H, Lunde P, Rasmussen K. Mitral flow derived Doppler indices of left ventricular diastolic function in a general population: the Tromsø study. Eur Heart J. 2000;21:1376–1386.

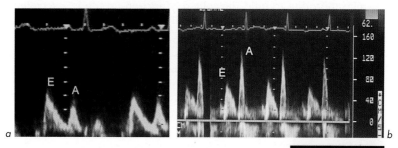

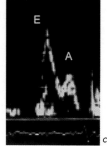

Figure 4.13 Mitral flow patterns on pulsed wave Doppler. **(a)** Normal. **(b)** Tall A-wave. **(c)** Tall E-wave.

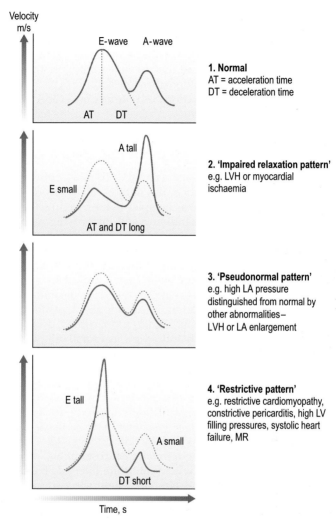

Figure 4.14 Mitral valve flow patterns. Normal pattern and patterns associated with different grades of LV diastolic dysfunction and some other conditions.

OTHER ECHO METHODS TO ASSESS DIASTOLIC FUNCTION

These include 'acoustic quantification' available on some echo machines. Using automatic border detection software, the endocardial border of the LV can be continuously outlined on a 4-chamber view. This can produce LV area/time and LV volume/time curves. Abnormalities of these diastolic filling parameters can be detected even when the mitral Doppler flow pattern is normal and this appears to be a sensitive technique to detect early diastolic dysfunction.

MEASUREMENT OF LA VOLUME

LA volume increases in LV diastolic dysfunction, due to chronically elevated LA pressure. LA volume can be measured from an apical 4-chamber view, at end-systole (on the still frame just before MV opens), using Simpson's method (Section 4.2).

LA volume should be indexed to body surface area (BSA). Normal is <34 mL/m^2 for both genders.

MYOCARDIAL TISSUE DOPPLER IMAGING (TDI)

During diastolic LV filling, the myocardial walls move outwards. The amplitude, pattern and velocity of this motion can be recorded using pulsed wave TDI (also known as Doppler tissue imaging, DTI). This is an important method of identifying and quantifying myocardial mechanics. Velocities measured by pulsed wave TDI have clinical and prognostic use. The velocity scale, wall filters and gain of the echo machine are adjusted to display the Doppler velocities of the movement of the myocardium, which are lower than intracavity blood flow velocities. These velocities are less dependent upon preload and are useful, in addition to Doppler transmitral flow, in evaluating diastolic function. Signals are recorded using pulsed wave Doppler in an apical 4-chamber view in a small sample volume of 2–3 mm positioned in the myocardium of the basal LV wall, about 1 cm from the mitral annulus. Signals may be recorded from the basal septum or basal lateral wall although the septal signals tend to be more reproducible. The velocity scale is decreased to a range of only around 0.2 m/s and the wall filters are reduced to obtain a well-defined signal. Some echo machines have a tissue Doppler setting that automatically makes these adjustments. Recordings are made at end expiration during normal quiet respiration.

The cardiac cycle can be divided into time intervals based upon mechanical events: filling and ejection. There are also isovolumic intervals before and after ejection. During ejection, there is a positive systolic myocardial wave towards the transducer (S_m or s′, S′). The filling period has 2 elements – E_m (or e′, E′) and A_m (or a′, A′) (Fig. 4.15). The pattern of myocardial motion is similar but inverted and lower in velocity compared to transmitral flows. When myocardial tissue Doppler velocities are recorded from the mitral annulus using an apical approach, there is a brief early velocity away from the transducer corresponding to early diastolic relaxation with a velocity of 8–12 cm/s. This is called the early myocardial velocity (E_m, or e′, E′). Following atrial contraction, a second velocity wave away from the apex is seen, the atrial myocardial velocity (A_m or a′, A′), usually 4–8 cm/s. The normal ratio of $E_m : A_m$ is over 1.0. A reduced $E_m : A_m$ ratio indicates impaired relaxation. The pattern of $E_m : A_m$ also helps to distinguish

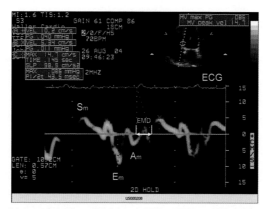

Figure 4.15 Myocardial tissue Doppler imaging (TDI). Apical 4-chamber view showing septal motion. *Sm,* systolic; *Em,* early; *Am,* atrial myocardial velocities; *EMD,* electro-mechanical delay.

normal LV filling from the pseudonormalization pattern seen in patients with moderate-to-severe diastolic dysfunction.

Approximate values for TDI-derived variables and IVRT are:

- E_m 10.3 ± 2.0 cm/s
- A_m 5.8 ± 1.6 cm/s
- E_m/A_m 2.1 ± 0.9
- IVRT 63 ± 11 ms

PULMONARY VENOUS FLOW

Pulmonary venous flow pattern, velocities and durations change with raised LA volume and pressure, due to LV diastolic dysfunction. Pulsed wave Doppler can be used to measure pulmonary venous flow in an apical 4-chamber view, with a 2–3 mm sample volume >5 mm (ideally 1–2 cm) into a pulmonary vein.

Although measurements can be obtained in >80% of adults (lower in the ICU setting), their quality is often affected by artefacts caused by LA wall motion. Figure 4.16 shows a normal pulmonary venous flow pattern.

ECHO METHOD TO ASSESS LV DIASTOLIC FUNCTION

The American Society of Echocardiography (ASE) and European Association of Echocardiography (EAE) (2009) have issued guidance for the assessment of LV diastolic function (Fig. 4.17). It is based upon 4 groups of echo measurements:

1. LA size. In diastolic LV dysfunction, LA enlargement is due to chronically raised LA pressure
2. Tissue Doppler imaging of LV

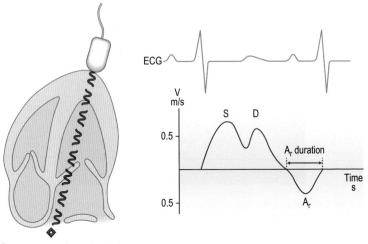

ECG

V
m/s

S   D

0.5

A_r duration

Time
s

0.5

A_r

◆ = sampling volume of pulsed wave
    Doppler in pulmonary vein

Figure 4.16 Pulmonary venous flow. Pulsed wave Doppler sampling volume placed in a pulmonary vein, 1–2 cm from orifice. *S*, systolic flow; *D*, diastolic flow; *Ar*, retrograde flow due to atrial contraction. Red arrow indicates Ar duration.

3. Transmitral flow by pulsed wave Doppler – to assess LV filling

4. Pulmonary venous flow by pulsed wave Doppler – changes in LA volume and pressure can impact pulmonary venous flow patterns, velocities and duration.

In the absence of other identifiable causes, increased LA size and abnormal LV TDI values suggest LV diastolic dysfunction. The MV and pulmonary venous flow patterns help to assess the severity.

Grading diastolic function appears to be prognostically important. Some studies suggest that, even in asymptomatic individuals (and after controlling for age, sex and LVEF), mild (grade I) diastolic dysfunction was associated with a 5-fold increase in 3-year and 5-year all-cause mortality, when compared with individuals with normal diastolic function. Mortality increased with increasing degree of diastolic dysfunction.

One should, however, sound a note of caution when diagnosing diastolic dysfunction, especially in older people. Assessment should consider factors such as age and heart rate (e.g. mitral E-wave, E : A ratio and E_m [e′] decrease with increasing heart rate). Specifically, many people aged >60 years, with no history or indicators of cardiovascular disease (e.g. no LVH), have an E : A ratio <1 and DT >200 ms and these can be considered normal for age.

Use echo in apical 4-chamber view to assess:

1 **LA volume** – using Simpson's method
  • measured in atrial diastole
  • normal <34 mL/m²
  • increased LA volume reflects increased
    LA pressure due to increased LV stiffness

AND

2 **Tissue doppler imaging (TDI)**
  • measure LV septal and lateral $E_m(e')$
  • normal LV septal E_m ≥8 cm/s
  • normal LV lateral E_m ≥10 cm/s

IF

Both
  • LA volume
  • TDI
  are normal

  • **Normal LV
    diastolic function**

  • enlarged LA
    +
  • normal TDI

  • **Normal or e.g.**
  • **Valvular abnormality**
    (e.g. mitral stenosis) or
  • **Athletic heart** or
  • **Constrictive pericarditis**

  • enlarged LA (≥34 mL/m²)
    +
  • abnormal TDI (septal E_m <8cm/s
    or lateral E_m <10 cm/s)

  • **LV diastolic dysfunction**
    To grade severity:

THEN

3 **Mitral flow**
  • measure E-wave, A-wave, E/A, DT

AND

4 **Pulmonary venous flow**
  • measure S-wave, D-wave, A_r, A_r duration

  *Grading of LV diastolic dysfunction

  Grade I – mild (impaired relaxation pattern)
  Grade II – moderate (pseudonormal pattern)
  Grade III – severe (restrictive pattern)

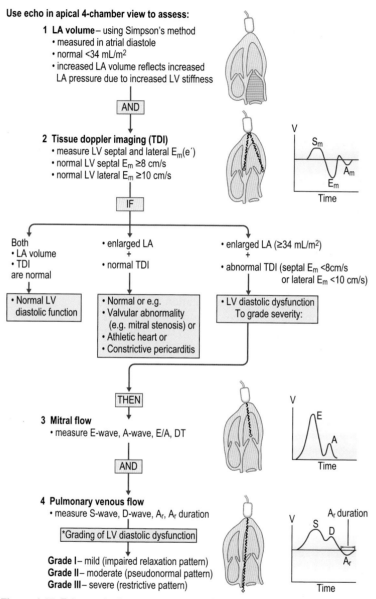

Figure 4.17 Echo method to assess LV diastolic function. *Em (or e′, E′)*, early myocardial velocity; *E*, mitral E-wave velocity; *A*, mitral A-wave velocity; *DT*, deceleration time; *Ar*, retrograde flow due to atrial contraction; *Ar–A*, duration of Ar minus duration of A-wave. *Grading of LV diastolic dysfunction is based upon:
Grade I (mild) – E/A <0.8, DT >200 ms, mean E/Em ≤8, Ar–A <0 ms.
Grade II (moderate) – E/A 0.8–1.5, DT 160–200 ms, mean E/Em 9–12, Ar–A ≥30 ms.
Grade III (severe) – E/A ≥2.0, DT <160 ms, mean E/Em ≥13, Ar–A ≥30 ms.
Based upon American Society of Echocardiography (ASE) and European Association of Echocardiography (EAE) guidance, 2009.

ATHLETIC HEART AND SCREENING BEFORE EXERCISE

Vigorous athletic training is associated with several physiological and biochemical adaptations that enable an increase in cardiac output. An increase in cardiac chamber size is fundamental to the generation of a sustained increase in cardiac output for prolonged periods. Echo studies have shown that the vast majority of athletes have modest cardiac enlargement although a small proportion exhibit substantial increases. Training results in compensated changes in cardiac anatomy, primarily of the LV, leading to the development of an 'athletic heart'. This does not occur in casual recreational athletes, as substantial training is needed for this to develop. The major determinants of cardiac morphological adaptation to training include body size (body surface area or height) and participation in certain endurance sports such as skiing, cycling, running and canoeing. Cardiac dimensions vary considerably amongst athletes, even when allowances are made for these variables, suggesting that genetic, endocrine and biochemical factors also influence heart size.

The type of athletic activity impacts on the nature of LV remodelling. In general, 2 main types of adaptation are recognized:

- LV chamber enlargement. Vigorous endurance training (e.g. long distance running/cycling/skiing/canoeing) leads to an endurance type of elevation in LV mass due to LV chamber enlargement and, to a lesser degree, an increase in wall thickness and mild LVH.
- LVH. Intense isotonic training (e.g. weight lifting) leads to a 'strength type' concentric LVH.

Note that many athletes use a combination of these endurance and strengthening training techniques, so these 'pure' categories of athletic heart are rare and most have a combination. Some people involved in intense competition have used anabolic steroid supplements, which can cause significant pathological LVH.

The clinical **echo** differentiation of athletic heart from other causes of LVH such as HCM (Table 4.4) can be difficult but may be helped by the following points:

- In general, in males with an athletic heart, LV posterior wall (LVPW) diastolic thickness is rarely over 13 mm (it may be 13–16 mm in approximately 2% of male athletes).
- The posterior wall thickness to LV diameter ratio remains normal.
- LVPW thickness of over 16 mm has not been reported due to athletic heart alone and should raise the possibility of HCM.
- The differentiation between athletic heart and pathological LVH is less difficult in female athletes, as LV wall thickness in elite female athletes is 6–12 mm (in the normal range) and so increased wall thickness is likely to be abnormal.
- Other ways to differentiate athletic heart from pathological hypertrophy include examining diastolic function using transmitral

Table 4.4 Echo features differentiating HCM from athletic heart

	HCM	Athletic heart
Clinical history	HCM family history	Endurance athlete
Effect of detraining	No effect	Regression of echo findings
LV systolic function	May be abnormal	Normal
LV diastolic function	Abnormal	Normal/supranormal
LVEDD	<4.5 cm	>5.5 cm
Interventricular septum thickness or LV posterior wall thickness in diastole	No limit	<1.6 cm

E : A ratios, tissue Doppler imaging for peak E_m wave velocity, which is high over the septum and lateral wall in athletes (over 8 cm/s), and tissue strain imaging.

Tests other than echo may be carried out. Measurement of maximum oxygen consumption during exercise (MVO_2) is useful and is supranormal in people with athletic hearts relative to people with HCM.

Screening and echo before exercise

Before undertaking competitive athletic activities in many countries, individuals are advised to undergo a general health evaluation. From the cardiovascular viewpoint, this means a full clinical history (e.g. of any cardiac symptoms and any family history of HCM or sudden death) and a full examination including BP, pulse and cardiovascular examination. Further investigation may include ECG, exercise ECG and echo. With no symptoms or family history and a normal examination, the chance of finding significant heart disease, likely to affect exercise capacity, is very low. Echo may, in these patients, have a low yield. **Echo** should be performed if there is:
- History of exertional syncope
- Family history of sudden cardiac death or HCM
- Murmur suggestive of HCM or AS.

Screening of athletes

In some countries, an echo is recommended for all professional athletes.

Screening for relevant conditions that may cause LVOTO (e.g. HOCM or AS) should be detected by clinical assessments. Disease of the proximal aorta or occult valve diseases are rare. Echo can, in some cases, identify the origin of both coronary arteries. This is important as anomalous origins of coronary arteries have been associated with sudden death during exercise.

Conditions increasing the risk of exercise that may be detected by echo

High/moderate risk:
- HOCM
- Aortic dilatation (e.g. Marfan's)
- Valvular AS (severe or moderate)
- Occult dilated cardiomyopathy
- PHT
- Anomalous origin of the coronary arteries.

Low risk:
- MV prolapse with mild MR
- Mild AS such as bicuspid AV with a Doppler gradient of under 36 mmHg
- Mild MS
- Mild PS
- Uncomplicated ASD
- Small restrictive VSD.

4.6 RIGHT HEART AND LUNGS

RIGHT VENTRICULAR (RV) FUNCTION

RV function plays a critical role in a number of congenital and acquired cardiac conditions. Accurate measurement of RV function is important in planning treatment and predicting prognosis. Until recently, RV function has attracted less attention than LV function. The main reasons have been a lack of understanding of its important role in the circulation and difficulties in assessing its function due to its complex anatomy.

Echo plays a role in assessing RV volume and function but is often used in combination with other modalities such as contrast ventriculography, radionuclide ventriculography, ultrafast CT and MRI. Even more accurate assessment can be made by the construction of RV pressure–volume loops (usually using data from cardiac catheterization).

Clinical importance of RV function

1. Myocardial infarction

RV dysfunction is well recognized in MI. Anterior MI is usually associated with persistent LV regional impairment and transient global RV impairment, whereas inferior MI is associated with persistent regional impairment in both ventricles. The haemodynamic responses to infarction differ in the RV and LV. In patients with

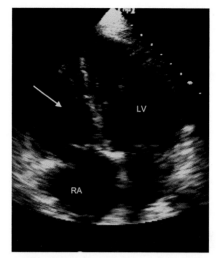

Figure 4.18 Dilated right ventricle (arrow) following acute right ventricular infarction. Apical 4-chamber view.

extensive RV infarction, cardiogenic shock is common and requires a different therapeutic approach from LV infarction (Fig. 4.18).

The degree of RV dysfunction can be used to assess prognosis in acute MI. RV ejection fraction (EF) is a useful indicator of outcome, and 2-year mortality is higher in patients with a low RV EF (<35%).

RV function is also important in predicting the prognosis in patients with VSD following MI. RV dysfunction is a major cause of cardiogenic shock and death in such patients.

2. Valvular heart disease (e.g. MS, PS)

RV function can play an important role in timing surgery.

3. Chronic lung disease causing PHT

RV function plays an important role in the long-term outcome of patients with chronic airflow limitation or pulmonary fibrosis. When such diseases are associated with PHT, RV dilatation and failure (leading to cor pulmonale), they have a poor outlook.

4. Septicaemic shock and post-cardiotomy shock

These are also associated with RV dysfunction, probably as a result of alterations in RV afterload and contractility.

5. Congenital heart disease before and after surgery (e.g. VSD, ASD, complex disease)

Assessment of RV function is of great importance. It is an important prognostic marker in patients with shunts (e.g. VSD, ASD) or complex conditions such as tetralogy of Fallot or transposition of the great arteries.

6. Pericardial effusion

RV diastolic collapse is an important echo indicator of cardiac tamponade.

Echo assessment of RV function

This is difficult because:

1. The RV has greater geometrical complexity than the LV.
2. The RV free wall is heavily trabeculated, making edge recognition difficult.
3. Overlap between RV and other cardiac chambers in some imaging modalities makes reliable volume measurement difficult.
4. The location of the RV directly under the sternum poses specific problems for echo (the ultrasound beam will not penetrate bone).
5. The assessment of the RV is especially difficult in people who have had previous thoracic surgery or have chronic lung disease. RV function studies are often vital for them.

Despite such limitations, **M-mode** and **2-D echo** are used to estimate RV size and function. The best echo views for the RV are usually:

- Subcostal 4-chamber
- Apical 4-chamber
- Parasternal long-axis, with transducer angulation to show RV inflow and outflow
- Parasternal short-axis at MV, papillary muscle and AV levels.

Estimates can be made of RV internal dimensions, wall thickness and EF. RV function is sensitive to myocardial contractility, preload and afterload but also to LV contractility, the contribution of the septum and to intrapericardial pressure. An analysis of RV function should take all these factors into account and EF *per se* may not be sensitive enough to these factors.

Right-sided failure is associated with a dilated, hypokinetic RV. If the RV is the same size or larger than the LV in all views, it is abnormal.

Note that even in the most experienced hands, adequate echo examination of the RV may be obtained in only approximately 50% of subjects.

Newer 3-D echo techniques (Section 5.4) have improved the assessment of RV structure and function.

PULMONARY HYPERTENSION

This is defined as an abnormal increase in PA pressure above:

- 30/20 mmHg (normal 25/10 mmHg) at rest
- Mean 25 mmHg at rest
- Mean 30 mmHg during exercise.

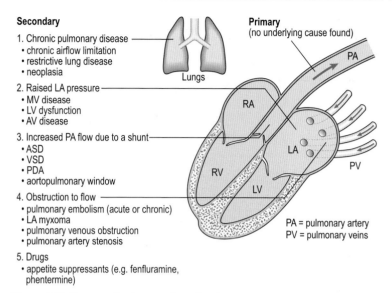

Secondary
1. Chronic pulmonary disease
   • chronic airflow limitation
   • restrictive lung disease
   • neoplasia
2. Raised LA pressure
   • MV disease
   • LV dysfunction
   • AV disease
3. Increased PA flow due to a shunt
   • ASD
   • VSD
   • PDA
   • aortopulmonary window
4. Obstruction to flow
   • pulmonary embolism (acute or chronic)
   • LA myxoma
   • pulmonary venous obstruction
   • pulmonary artery stenosis
5. Drugs
   • appetite suppressants (e.g. fenfluramine, phentermine)

Primary
(no underlying cause found)

PA = pulmonary artery
PV = pulmonary veins

Figure 4.19 Causes of pulmonary hypertension.

The severity of PHT may be categorized as:
• Mild: PA systolic pressure <40 mmHg at rest
• Moderate: PA systolic pressure 40–70 mmHg at rest
• Severe: PA systolic pressure >70 mmHg at rest (mean PA pressure >40 mmHg).

In people aged over 50 years, PHT is the third most frequent cardiovascular problem after coronary artery disease and systemic hypertension.

Echo is useful in assessing the underlying cause (Fig. 4.19) and severity of PHT (Fig. 4.20), but echo examination can be technically more difficult since many of these patients have underlying lung disease. This is especially true if the lungs are hyperinflated or there is pulmonary fibrosis.

The echo features of PHT

M-mode
• Abnormal M-mode of the PV leaflets with absent A-wave or mid-systolic notch
• Dilated RV with normal LV
• Abnormal IVS motion ('right ventricularization' of IVS)
• Underlying cause, e.g. MS (PA systolic pressure is an index of severity).

2-D echo
• Dilated PA (e.g. parasternal short-axis view at aortic level). The PA diameter should normally not be greater than the aortic diameter

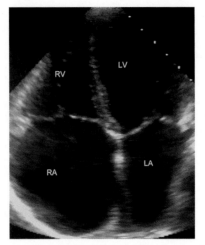

Figure 4.20 Pulmonary hypertension. Dilated right atrium and right ventricle in apical 4-chamber view.

- RV dilatation and/or hypertrophy
- RA dilatation
- Abnormal IVS motion
- Underlying cause, e.g. MV or AV disease, ASD, VSD, LV dysfunction.

Doppler

This is the best method to assess PA systolic pressure using TR velocity (as described in Chapter 3), or short PA acceleration time (AT, the time from onset of pulmonary arterial flow to peak velocity) as a surrogate of PHT. Pulmonary AT >140 ms indicates normal PA systolic pressure, AT <90 ms indicates PA systolic pressure >70 mmHg (severe PHT).

PULMONARY EMBOLISM

Pulmonary embolism (PE) refers to the situation when a mass, usually a blood clot (thrombus) travels in the bloodstream and lodges in the pulmonary arterial system. The origin of the thrombus is usually a systemic vein, often in the legs, pelvis or abdomen. Materials other than thrombus may embolize and include tumours, fat or air. PE is a very common condition and microemboli are found in up to 60% of autopsies, but are diagnosed less frequently in life. Up to 10% of clinically detected PEs are fatal. After PE, lung tissue is ventilated with air but not perfused with blood. This leads to impaired gas exchange and hypoxia (a reduction in the amount of oxygen in the blood). After a few hours, the area of lung involved may collapse and subsequently infarct. The haemodynamic effect of PE is a rise in PA pressure and a fall in cardiac output. Echo may help in the diagnosis. There may be no obvious underlying cause, but the thrombus that may lead to PE can form as a result of:

- Sluggish blood flow
- Local injury
- Venous compression
- Hypercoagulable state.

Risk factors for PE

- Immobility
- Prolonged bed-rest
- Lower limb and pelvic fractures
- Malignancy
- Debilitating systemic diseases, e.g. heart failure
- Pregnancy and childbirth
- Post-surgery, especially abdominal or pelvic
- Inherited hypercoagulable states, e.g. factor V Leiden and deficiency of protein S, protein C or anti-thrombin III
- Smoking
- Excess oestrogen, e.g. oral contraceptive pill.

Clinical features of PE

There are varied presentations, depending on the size of the PE and the extent of obstruction of the pulmonary circulation. PEs usually present with pleuritic chest pain, dyspnoea, haemoptysis or haemodynamic collapse if there is acute massive PE. The effects of the PE relate to its size and the degree of obstruction in the pulmonary circulation.

There are 4 distinct presentations with different clinical and echo features:

1. **Silent PE**. Many small PEs are not detected clinically.
2. **Small/medium PE**. PE in a terminal pulmonary vessel.
   - Pleuritic chest pain and breathlessness. Haemoptysis in 30% often 3 days or more after PE. May present in a subtle non-specific way with unexplained breathlessness or cough or new-onset AF.
   - Tachypnoea, pleural rub, coarse crackles over area. Fever. Cardiovascular examination may be normal.
   - There may be a blood-stained pleural effusion.
   - Chest X-ray often normal.
   - ECG shows sinus tachycardia, AF, right heart strain if medium-sized PE.

- Blood tests show raised fibrin degradation products or D-dimer.
- Other tests may be useful in diagnosis including ultrasound of pelvis and legs, V/Q scan, spiral CT, MRI.
- **Echo** is usually normal with small PEs. With medium PEs, there may be some echo features of right heart dilatation.

3. **Massive PE**. Rarer. Presents with sudden collapse due to obstruction of RVOT because PE has lodged in main PA.
   - Severe central chest pain (due to myocardial ischaemia caused by reduced coronary arterial flow).
   - May result in shock, syncope due to a sudden reduction in cardiac output, or death.
   - Tachycardia, tachypnoea, hypotension, peripheral shut-down, haemodynamic collapse, raised JVP with a prominent 'a' wave, RV heave, gallop rhythm, widely split second heart sound.
   - Chest X-ray shows pulmonary oligaemia with prominence of main pulmonary trunk in hila.
   - ECG shows sinus tachycardia, RA dilatation, RV strain, right axis deviation, new partial or complete RBBB; there may be AF, and T-wave inversion in right chest leads. S1 Q3 T3 pattern is rare.
   - Pulmonary angiography or spiral CT may show PE.
   - **Echo** shows a vigorous LV, dilated RA and RV, raised PASP assessed from TR if obstruction above the level of PV. PE may be seen in RVOT.

4. **Multiple recurrent PEs**. Gradual obstruction of regions of the pulmonary arterial circulation.
   - This may lead to progressive breathlessness over weeks or months due to gradual obstruction of regions of the PA circulation. May present non-specifically with weakness, angina, palpitations or exertional syncope.
   - On examination, there are physical signs of PHT due to multiple occlusions of the pulmonary vascular bed with signs of RV overload with an RV heave and loud P_2.
   - Chest X-ray may be normal.
   - V/Q scan shows multiple mismatched defects; leg and pelvic ultrasound may show abnormality.
   - **Echo** shows features of PHT with dilated RV and RA and raised PASP.

The echo findings in PE relate to the size of the embolism and the degree of obstruction of the pulmonary circulation. Important points are:
- A normal echo does not exclude PE (this is particularly the case with small PEs).

- If there is pre-existing cardiovascular disease, this must be factored into the echo findings.
- Massive PE. There is a right heart pressure and volume overload pattern with RV dilatation and possibly failure and RA dilatation.
- TR may occur due to increased right heart pressures.
- With medium-sized PE, there may be milder right heart dilatation and TR.
- LV assessment is essential. An inferior MI with RV infarction may cause similar echo features of a dilated right heart, but there will be normal PASP, unlike the situation with PE where the PASP will be raised.
- RV pressures rarely exceed 60–70 mmHg. If the pressure is over 70 mmHg in PE, the differential diagnosis includes acute on chronic PE or PE on the background of PHT.

Occasionally, it is possible to see that there is a PE in the proximal PA. Sometimes, a PE 'in transit' may be seen, either caught in the TV apparatus or sometimes intraoperatively during TOE. On contrast echo, a right-to-left shunt via a patent foramen ovale (PFO) may be seen if the RA pressures increase and there may be bowing of the interatrial septum from right to left.

Echo features of a poorer prognosis with PE include:
- Significant right heart dilatation
- RV systolic dysfunction
- PE in transit.

Management of PE

- Acute treatment – resuscitation, high-concentration oxygen, analgesia, bedrest, fluids, inotropic support, intensive care
- Prevention of further PEs – anticoagulation (e.g. intravenous heparin then oral warfarin or other anticoagulant, usually for at least 6 months) or occasionally physical methods (e.g. insertion of a filter in the IVC above the level of the renal veins) if recurrent PEs or inability to take anticoagulants
- Dissolution of PE – thrombolytic therapy, for example, intravenous streptokinase or tissue plasminogen activator (tPA)
- Surgery – removal of PE is rarely needed, if massive.

4.7 LONG-AXIS FUNCTION

Ventricular systole involves longitudinal (long-axis) as well as circumferential (short-axis) shortening. Long-axis function gives important information about normal cardiac physiology and disease states. This can be assessed using several echo techniques, including M-mode, tissue Doppler imaging and strain/strain rate analysis of myocardial deformation (see also Section 7.9).

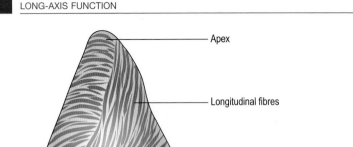

Apex

Longitudinal fibres

Circumferential (found in subendocardial
fibres   and subepicardial layers)

Mitral valve
orifice

Figure 4.21 Schematic representation of the arrangement of fibres of left ventricle.

ECHO ASSESSMENT OF LONG-AXIS FUNCTION

The LV (Fig. 4.21) and RV long-axes run from the apex (which is fixed relative to the chest wall) to the base of the heart (which is taken as the MV and TV rings). Function of separate parts can be examined (e.g. LV and RV free walls, IVS). Long-axis measurements are made using M-mode or Doppler echo. It is important to look at amplitude, velocity and timing of long-axis changes.

M-mode can be used to assess LV long-axis function by assessing mitral annular plane systolic excursion (MAPSE) and RV systolic function by assessing tricuspid annular plane systolic excursion (TAPSE) (Fig. 4.22, M-mode lines 1 and 3, respectively). The annular systolic velocities can also be measured – mitral annular systolic velocity (MASV) and tricuspid annular systolic velocity (TASV). Although normal values have not yet been confirmed in large population studies, the following reflect the approximate lower limit of normal long-axis LV and RV function:

- MAPSE   1.0 cm
- MASV   10 cm/s
- LV longitudinal systolic strain   −20%
- TAPSE   1.7 cm
- TASV   10 cm/s
- RV longitudinal systolic strain   −30%

Strain is the percentage change in a chamber dimension relative to its initial dimension.

These measurements are influenced by factors such as age, respiration and ultrasound beam angulation.

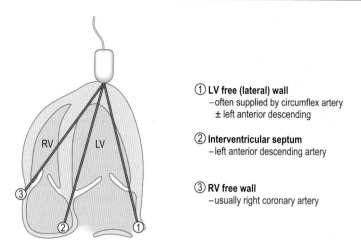

Figure 4.22 Long-axis function. M-mode study of movement of atrioventricular rings towards the apex.

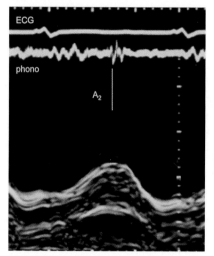

Figure 4.23 Long-axis function. M-mode showing movement of the mitral valve ring (left ventricle free wall side) towards the apex during systole. An ECG and phonocardiogram are recorded to allow timing of events, such as aortic valve closure (A_2).

Long-axis contribution to normal physiology (Figs. 4.22, 4.23)

1. Ejection fraction
Long-axis function plays a role in maintaining normal EF and changes in LV cavity shape.

2. Blood flow into atria
During ventricular systole, the MV and TV rings move towards the cardiac apex, increasing the capacity of the 2 atria as their

floor moves downwards. Atrial volumes increase (and pressure falls), drawing blood into the atria from the caval and pulmonary veins.

3. Early diastolic flow

The MV moves backwards towards the LA during early diastolic forward blood flow into the LV. Effectively, blood that was in the LA finds itself in the LV as the MV ring has moved backwards around it. LV volume has increased without blood actually moving with respect to the apex and chest wall! This is not detectable on Doppler. This and a similar effect during atrial systole account for 10–15% of LV stroke volume and 20% of RV.

The LA is not a passive structure. During ventricular systole, the LA is subject to external work from the ventricle and this is transferred back to the LV during early diastole and coupled to blood flow.

4. Atrial systole

Atrial blood volume falls during atrial systole. The lateral and back walls of the atria are fixed to the mediastinum and the dominant mechanism by which their volume falls is by movement of the AV rings away from the ventricular apex.

Long-axis function in disease

1. Ventricular function

Long-axis function gives a good estimate of the EF of both ventricles. This is useful when an apical 4-chamber view can be taken and parasternal views are difficult (e.g. in a severely ill, ventilated patient in the ICU).

Regional reduction in long-axis function is common after acute MI. These defects correlate with fixed defects on myocardial perfusion imaging (e.g. thallium).

After MV replacement, long-axis function is reduced, but not after MV repair or in MS. This does not occur consistently after cardiopulmonary bypass for other reasons and is likely to reflect loss of papillary muscle function.

In restrictive LV disease, long-axis amplitude is low even with a normal LV size at end-diastole.

2. Coronary artery disease and ischaemia

Long-axis function provides a remarkably sensitive, non-invasive assessment of ischaemia. This may be due to the fact that a significant proportion of longitudinal muscle fibres are located in the subendocardium. Long-axis function is often asynchronous in coronary disease (e.g. chronic stable angina) and segmental in distribution. Onset of contraction is often delayed. This effect may explain the 'abnormal relaxation' pattern of LV diastolic dysfunction seen with ageing (where the early E-wave on Doppler is reduced or absent and the A-wave increased).

3. Activation abnormalities
Long-axis function is sensitive to activation abnormalities possibly due to subendocardial location of fibres. Abnormalities occur in RBBB and LBBB. This allows assessment of the effects of abnormal activation, especially in patients with severe ventricular disease and of different pacing modes in patients with heart failure.

4. LVH
LV diastolic function is abnormal in LVH even when short-axis systolic function is not. Long-axis function is often abnormal.

5. Atrial function
Restoration of atrial mechanical function after cardioversion of AF (Section 7.2) can be demonstrated by long-axis function (RA is restored more rapidly than LA). Contraction of pectinate muscles causes movement of the atrioventricular ring. This is the earliest consequence of atrial mechanical activity.

4.8 PERICARDIAL DISEASE

The pericardium is the sac that surrounds the heart and is made up of the outer fibrous pericardium and the inner serous pericardium, which has an outer parietal layer (attached to the fibrous sac) and an inner visceral layer (or epicardium, attached to the heart) (Fig. 4.24).

There is a potential pericardial space between the 2 layers of serous pericardium normally containing a small volume (<50 mL) of pericardial fluid.

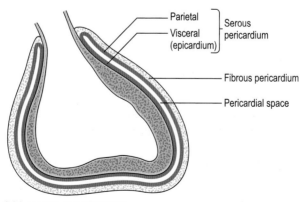

Figure 4.24 Layers of pericardium.

Echo is the most effective method to assess many of the pathological changes that may affect the pericardium causing an increase in pericardial fluid (pericardial effusion), cardiac tamponade or constrictive pericarditis. The normal fibrous pericardium is highly echo-reflective and appears echo-bright. Fluid in the pericardial space is poorly reflective and appears black. Some individuals may have a pericardial fat pad or cyst (see Section 6.1).

1. PERICARDIAL EFFUSION

A pericardial effusion may be composed of serous fluid, blood or, rarely, pus (when the person is very seriously ill).

Causes of pericardial effusion

- Infection – viral, bacterial including tuberculosis, fungal
- Malignancy
- Heart failure
- Post MI – Dressler's syndrome
- Cardiac trauma or surgery
- Uraemia
- Autoimmune – rheumatoid arthritis, SLE, scleroderma
- Inflammation – amyloid, sarcoid
- Hypothyroidism
- Drugs – phenylbutazone, penicillins, procainamide, hydralazine, isoniazid
- Aortic dissection
- Radiation
- Idiopathic.

M-mode and **2-D echo** are the most important methods to assess pericardial effusion (Figs. 4.25, 4.26). On M-mode, using a parasternal long-axis view, the echo-free pericardial effusion may be below the LV posterior wall or above the anterior wall of the RV. On 2-D imaging, the effusion can be seen as an echo-free space surrounding the heart. The effusion may be throughout the pericardial space or loculated in certain regions only.

Differentiation between pericardial and pleural effusion can be made on 2-D or M-mode (although the 2 may co-exist) (Fig. 4.27). Unlike pleural effusion, the echo-free space of pericardial effusion terminates at the AV groove and does not extend beyond the level of the descending aorta.

Estimation of the volume of pericardial effusion present can be made by echo. This can be done qualitatively on M-mode or 2-D by the depth to the echo-free space around the heart. A more accurate method is to use the planimetry (area estimation) function present

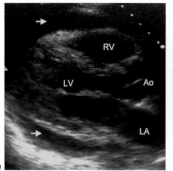
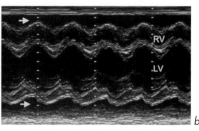

Figure 4.25 Pericardial effusion. **(a)** Parasternal long-axis view showing effusion anterior to right ventricle and posterior to left ventricle (arrows). **(b)** M-mode showing effusion (arrows).

Figure 4.26 Pericardial effusion. **(a)** Parasternal short-axis view at mitral valve level showing effusion (arrows). **(b)** Magnified subcostal view showing fibrin strands (arrow) in the effusion (PE).

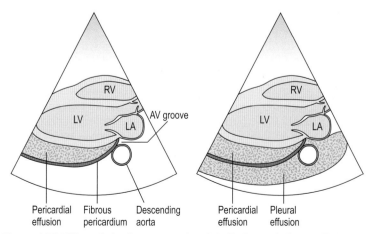

Figure 4.27 Differentiation between pericardial effusion and pleural effusion on 2-D echo.

on most echo machine computers. A still image of an apical 4-chamber view is taken and the following measurements are made:

1. A tracing around the pericardium (from which the computer calculates the combined volumes of the heart and pericardium)
2. A tracing around the heart (which gives the volume of the heart).

   The volume of the effusion is obtained by subtracting these volumes.

2. CARDIAC TAMPONADE

This is a dangerous situation in which cardiac function is impaired due to external pressure upon the heart (e.g. due to fluid accumulation or pericardial constriction). Tamponade may result from a large volume of pericardial effusion or a rapidly forming small volume of effusion that causes pressure on the heart (very large effusions can form without causing tamponade if the pericardial sac has time to stretch to accommodate the fluid).

Clinical features of tamponade

- Tachycardia (heart rate >100)
- Hypotension (systolic BP <100 mmHg) with a small pulse volume
- Pulsus paradoxus of >10 mmHg (an exaggeration of the normal small [<5 mmHg] fall in systolic BP during inspiration)
- Raised JVP with a prominent 'X' systolic descent. The JVP may not fall as normal on inspiration or infrequently may paradoxically rise (Kussmaul's paradox).

Remember: Tamponade is a **clinical** diagnosis. Echo can provide supportive evidence of it.

Echo features of tamponade

- Large volume pericardial effusion.
- RA and/or RV diastolic collapse. Both are sensitive to tamponade. After relief of tamponade by drainage of the effusion, RV diastolic collapse soon reverses. Diastolic RA collapse does not do so as quickly and may be the more sensitive indicator of tamponade.
- Doppler features are of exaggerated changes in transmitral and transtricuspid flows normally seen with inspiration and expiration and changes in flow patterns of the superior vena cava (SVC).

Echo may aid in safely performing therapeutic echo-guided needle aspiration of pericardial fluid (pericardiocentesis) to relieve the tamponade, which may be life saving. Echo can help to locate the site and extent of fluid collection and assess the success of the procedure.

3. ACUTE PERICARDITIS

This is inflammation of the pericardium and has several causes. There may be associated pericardial effusion. The clinical features vary widely. Some people may be relatively asymptomatic, whilst other people may experience a severe illness with inflammation extending to the myocardium (myopericarditis) with haemodynamic collapse. Acute pericarditis may be recurrent.

Clinical features of acute pericarditis

• Chest pain that is retrosternal and may be referred to the shoulders or neck. The pain is worsened by respiration, usually by taking a deep breath (pleuritic chest pain) and by movement. The pain is often worse on lying flat and improved by sitting forwards.
• Fever, especially when pericarditis is due to viral or bacterial infection, myocardial infarction or rheumatic fever.
• Malaise.
• Pericardial friction rub. This is a scratching/crunching superficial sound. It has been described as the sound made by the feet when 'walking on snow'.

Causes of pericarditis

• Idiopathic
• Viral infection (e.g. Coxsackie)
• Myocardial infarction – acute or 1 month to 1 year later (Dressler's syndrome)
• Uraemia – in the terminal stages of renal failure and may be asymptomatic
• Malignancy – especially carcinoma of bronchus or breast, Hodgkin's lymphoma, leukaemia, malignant melanoma
• Tuberculosis – low-grade fever (especially in the evening) with malaise, weight loss and features of acute pericarditis (pericardial aspiration may be needed to diagnose)
• Bacterial – purulent pericarditis with pneumonia (e.g. *Staphylococcus aureus*, *Haemophilus influenzae* or septicaemia); often fatal; treatment is with antibiotics with or without surgical drainage
• Trauma
• Radiotherapy – only if the heart is not fully shielded.

Investigations

The ECG is diagnostic showing ST elevation with a saddle-shaped concave upward ST segment (Fig. 4.28). The inflammatory markers (erythrocyte sedimentation rate [ESR] and C-reactive protein) and white blood cell count are elevated. Cardiac enzymes and troponins may be elevated if there is associated myocarditis.

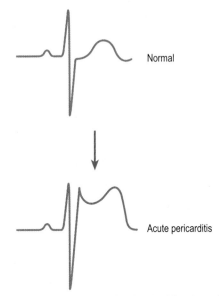

Figure 4.28 ECG in acute pericarditis showing 'saddle-shaped' ST segment elevation (arrow).

Treatment

Non-steroidal anti-inflammatory drugs and steroids are given if the pericarditis is severe or recurrent.

An **echo** is often requested for individuals who clinically have acute pericarditis.

Echo features of acute pericarditis

- The echo may be normal with no pathognomonic features in uncomplicated viral pericarditis
- There may be a pericardial effusion
- Associated features (e.g. regional wall motion abnormalities with acute myocardial infarction)
- 'Thickened' pericardium.

Use of echo in acute pericarditis

- Aids in diagnosis of underlying aetiology
- Detects complications such as effusion, myopericarditis, and systolic and diastolic ventricular dysfunction
- Associated pericardial effusion
- Regional wall motion abnormalities
- Tumour detection

- Differential diagnosis from conditions with similar presentation (e.g. vegetations and MR in a patient with fever, systolic murmur or rub due to infective endocarditis)
- In people with chest pain within 12 hours of an acute coronary syndrome to differentiate myocardial damage (wall motion abnormalities) from pericarditis.

4. CONSTRICTIVE PERICARDITIS

In this condition, the relatively flexible fibrous pericardium becomes more rigid, due to fibrosis or calcification, limiting the diastolic expansion of the ventricles and reducing diastolic filling.

Causes of constrictive pericarditis

- Tuberculosis
- Connective tissue disorders
- Malignancy
- Trauma and post-cardiac surgery
- Uraemia
- Other infection – bacterial, viral
- Idiopathic.

Echo is important in the diagnosis and assessment of constrictive pericarditis. It is helpful to try to understand the underlying physiological mechanisms.

When the heart is encased in the rigid pericardium, the ability of all the cardiac chambers to change volumes during the normal cardiac cycle is affected. This affects the pressures, flows and volumes in all parts of the heart and its venous and arterial connections. In constrictive pericarditis, the total volume of the 4 cardiac chambers is relatively fixed. An increase in the volume of one chamber occurs at the expense of the other chambers. This is known as interdependence.

During normal respiration, for example, the fall in intrathoracic pressure during inspiration increases venous return to the right heart. In constrictive pericarditis, because of interdependence, increased right heart volumes (RA and RV) limit and decrease left heart volumes. (This is compounded by a reduced return of blood to the left heart from the lungs with lower intrathoracic pressure.) Starling's mechanism of the heart states, in simple terms, that in a normal heart, increased stretch of a cardiac chamber results in a greater ejection force and increased stroke volume – i.e. more blood into a chamber results in more blood out. Decreased left heart volumes lead to reduced stroke volume into the aorta. This is one factor in causing the marked fall in systolic blood pressure during inspiration (pulsus paradoxus) that is seen in constrictive pericarditis.

These physiological changes can help us to understand the echo findings in constrictive pericarditis:

- Ventricular filling is prematurely curtailed (in early or mid-diastole), limiting the diastolic expansion of the ventricles and reducing diastolic filling
- End-diastolic LV and RV volumes are decreased, with a consequent reduction in stroke volume
- Pressures increase in all 4 cardiac chambers and their venous connections
- Raised RA and LA pressures and limited filling cause flow to the RV and LV to be of short duration and high velocity
- Because the maximum volume of the heart is fixed, an increase in volume of the right heart limits the increase in volume of the left heart and vice versa (interdependence)
- The heart is relatively isolated from normal respiratory changes in intrathoracic pressure, but its venous and arterial connections (which are outside the pericardium) are not. This leads to abnormal cardiac filling patterns with respiration and affects stroke volume and blood pressure (by Starling's mechanism, as described above).

Echo features of constrictive pericarditis

M-mode and 2-D echo

- Thickened pericardium. This is difficult to quantify and often tends to be overestimated. The normal pericardium is highly echogenic and appears bright. The degree of this depends upon the gain settings on the echo machine. On M-mode, the thickened pericardium appears as a dark thick echo line or as multiple separated parallel lines.
- Calcified pericardium – localized or generalized.
- Abnormal septal motion, especially end-diastolic (exaggerated anterior motion, 'septal bounce').
- Dilated IVC due to raised systemic venous pressure.
- Abnormal LV filling pattern – LV only expands in early diastole. Difficult to recognize in real-time. On M-mode this appears as mid- and late-diastolic flattening of LVPW motion.
- Premature MV closure – due to raised LV diastolic pressure.
- Premature diastolic opening of the PV with increased RV end-diastolic pressure.

Doppler

Abnormal MV flow pattern reflecting abnormal diastolic LV filling of a 'restrictive pattern'.

- Increase in early diastolic velocity (E-wave large)
- Rapid deceleration
- Very small A-wave compared with E (E : A ratio >1.5)
- Short pressure half-time of mitral and tricuspid valve flow

- Exaggerated respiratory variation of MV flow (decreased E-wave by >25% on inspiration) or TV flow (decreased E-wave by >25% on expiration)
- Abnormal hepatic venous and pulmonary venous flow patterns
- Prominent systolic 'X' descent of SVC flow.

It can be difficult to diagnose constrictive pericarditis accurately on echo. It is particularly hard to distinguish from restrictive cardiomyopathy or a restrictive myocardial function pattern due to myocardial infiltration (Table 4.5). Cardiac MRI and direct pressure

Table 4.5 Echo differentiation of constrictive pericarditis from restrictive cardiomyopathy

	Constrictive pericarditis	Restrictive cardiomyopathy
Pericardium	Thickened >4 mm (can be difficult to assess) and/or calcified	Normal
LV size and thickness	Normal	LVH, small LV cavity
LV systolic function	Normal	May be abnormal
LV diastolic function	Normal	Abnormal
LA and RA volumes	Normal	Increased
Interventricular septal motion	Respiratory shift	Normal
Transmitral flow pattern	Respiratory variation in IVRT and E-wave velocity E>A, E : A ratio>1.5	No significant respiratory variation in IVRT and E-wave velocity E<A – early disease E>A – late disease
Hepatic venous flow	Expiratory diastolic flow reversal	Inspiratory diastolic flow reversal
Pulmonary venous flow	Systolic flow dominant	Diastolic flow dominant
Pulmonary artery systolic pressure	Mild elevation (35–40 mmHg)	Moderate to severe elevation (≥60 mmHg)
Myocardial tissue Doppler imaging (TDI)	Normal or increased velocities (e.g. E_m, e')	Reduced velocities (e.g. E_m, e')
LV septal E_m, e'	≥7 cm/s	<7 cm/s
E : E_m ratio	<15	>15

A, *MV A-wave velocity;* E, *MV E-wave velocity;* E_m *(or e'), early myocardial velocity by TDI;* IVRT, *isovolumic relaxation time;* LA, *left atrium;* LV, *left ventricle;* LVH, *left ventricular hypertrophy;* RA, *right atrium.*

measurements in catheterization studies may be needed to make the diagnosis.

4.9 DEVICE THERAPY FOR HEART FAILURE – CARDIAC RESYNCHRONIZATION THERAPY

There have been advances in the management of heart failure. Implantable electrical device therapy has become an option for some patients. Patients with heart failure may have poor co-ordination of the electrical activation (known as *electrical dyssynchrony*) and of the systolic and diastolic function of the LV and RV (known as *mechanical dyssynchrony*). They may have other problems affecting cardiac output, such as MR.

Cardiac resynchronization therapy (CRT) is a technique of simultaneous biventricular pacing that aims to improve the haemodynamic situation. CRT has added to the treatment options for patients, especially those with severe, drug-refractory and drug-optimized heart failure. Several large international studies have suggested benefit – e.g. MIRACLE (Multicenter InSync Randomized Clinical Evaluation), COMPANION (Comparison of Medical Therapy, Pacing, and Defibrillation in Heart Failure), CARE-HF (CArdiac Resynchronization-Heart Failure) and EchoCRT (Echocardiography Guided Cardiac Resynchronization Therapy). CRT is not suitable for all patients with heart failure, so methods have to be devised to select potential responders. It was hoped that echo may play a role in the selection of patients for CRT, but its role seems particularly helpful in optimizing therapy and monitoring progress.

How is CRT carried out?

CRT involves the implantation in the upper chest of an electrical pulse generator (pacemaker) device from which 3 pacing leads descend via veins into the heart (Figs. 4.29, 4.30). Leads are placed into the RA, RV and LV (the latter usually via the coronary sinus). These CRT pacing (CRT-P) devices are used to improve cardiac function by resynchronizing atrial, RV and LV function. Some devices also include a cardioverter-defibrillator function (these are known as CRT-D devices) and evidence suggests that these reduce mortality from VT and VF. Some devices also allow an estimation of thoracic impedance with changes in the degree of pulmonary interstitial fluid, which may give the patient or doctor an early indication of the development of pulmonary oedema.

Echo can be used to assess ventricular systolic and diastolic function (e.g. LVEF) and look for evidence of dyssynchrony and other features in heart failure, such as MR.

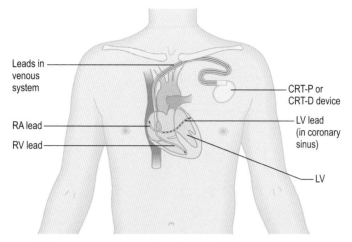

Leads in venous system

RA lead

RV lead

CRT-P or CRT-D device

LV lead (in coronary sinus)

LV

Figure 4.29 Cardiac resynchronization therapy (CRT) using a pacemaker (CRT-P) or a defibrillator (CRT-D).

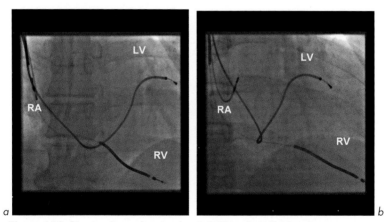

Figure 4.30 Chest radiographs showing 3 CRT leads in the heart.
(a) Antero-posterior and **(b)** right anterior oblique projections. The LV lead is in the coronary sinus.

Abnormal electrical activation and mechanical dyssynchrony in heart failure

The QRS complex of the ECG represents the vector sum of the electrical forces within the ventricular myocardium with time. Normal electrical activity propagates through the myocardial Purkinje network (Fig. 4.31). In damaged myocardium, conduction is impaired, changing the velocity and direction of electrical propagation and causing abnormal electrical activity. Abnormal ventricular depolarization generates regions of delayed and early ventricular

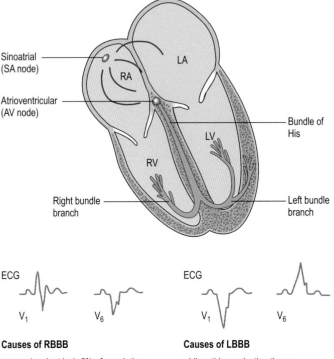

Causes of RBBB

- normal variant in 1–5% of population
- idiopathic conducting tissue disease/fibrosis
- congenital heart disease – ASD, VSD, PS, tetralogy of Fallot
- myocardial disease – cardiomyopathy
- coronary artery disease – acute MI
- pulmonary disease – cor pulmonale
- recurrent multiple PEs
- acute PE
- drugs and electrolyte abnormalities – class IA drugs, hypokalaemia
- RV surgery

Causes of LBBB

- idiopathic conducting tissue disease/fibrosis
- myocardial disease – cardiomyopathy
- coronary artery disease – acute MI, severe multi-vessel disease
- LVOT – AS
- LVH – hypertension

Figure 4.31 Myocardial conduction system – Purkinje network.

contraction causing dyssynchronized mechanical activity and impairing systolic and diastolic function.

In heart failure, there may be:

- Interventricular dyssynchrony – poor co-ordination of activation of LV relative to RV
- Intraventricular dyssynchrony – delayed activation of one LV region relative to another.

Abnormal depolarization is manifest on the ECG as QRS prolongation (bundle branch block, BBB). The pattern may be of left (LBBB), right

(RBBB) or non-specific intraventricular conduction delay. The normal QRS duration is under 120 ms. There is a direct relationship between QRS duration and ejection fraction and a good correlation between QRS duration and interventricular mechanical dyssynchrony has been demonstrated. RBBB may be a normal finding in up to 5% of the population. LBBB is pathological. Bundle branch block occurs in about 20% of the heart failure population, but in over 35% of patients with severe heart failure, and bundle branch block is a strong independent predictor of mortality.

Does echo play a role in patient selection for CRT?

The selection of patients with heart failure who may benefit from CRT remains complex. A number of large clinical studies have addressed this question but only some used echo measures of dyssynchrony in patient selection (e.g. in CARE-HF, where patients with a QRS of 120–149 ms made up 11% of the total in the study, and in EchoCRT).

It appears that QRS duration, especially with LBBB pattern, remains the main selection criterion for CRT. Patients with QRS durations >150 ms are more likely to respond than those with QRS durations of 130–150 ms. Echo assessment is not routinely needed in these individuals for selection prior to CRT, although echo is of benefit in assessing baseline measures (e.g. LV volumes and systolic function, degree of MR, some echo measures of mechanical dyssynchrony, etc.), to optimize CRT and to assess response to treatment. In the EchoCRT study, CRT was not found to be of benefit (and may be associated with adverse outcomes) in people with symptomatic heart failure, LVEF ≤35% and QRS duration <130 ms, with or without echo evidence of dyssynchrony.

In people with shorter QRS durations (e.g. 130–150 ms), echo measures of dyssynchrony may have some role in selecting potential CRT responders.

Echo in selection for CRT

* QRS duration >150 ms – echo assessment of mechanical dyssynchrony not needed
* QRS duration <130 ms – CRT not beneficial or may be harmful, even if echo evidence of dyssynchrony (EchoCRT study)
* QRS duration 130–150 ms – uncertain and echo assessment of dyssynchrony may be of some benefit (120–149 ms in CARE-HF study).

A beneficial response to CRT was initially considered to result in part from resynchronization of interventricular dyssynchrony (dyssynchrony between LV and RV). QRS duration alone, however, does not always predict good response to CRT. About 20–30% of patients fail to respond to CRT despite prolonged QRS. Evidence suggests that *LV intraventricular dyssynchrony is a more useful predictor of response to CRT than interventricular dyssynchrony*. Patients with a wider QRS complex have a higher likelihood of LV dyssynchrony but over 30% of patients with wide QRS lack LV dyssynchrony. This 30% may partially explain a similar percentage of non-responders in the studies. These observations resulted in studies evaluating different echo parameters to detect LV dyssynchrony and predict response to CRT.

Echo techniques have thus been developed to assess mechanical dyssynchrony with the aim of identifying potential responders to CRT. Echo can also measure LVEF and assess severity of MR in heart failure.

Aims of CRT

• Resynchronization of intraventricular contraction
• Resynchronization of interventricular contraction
• Optimization of atrioventricular co-ordination
• Reduction in MR
• Haemodynamic improvement
• Reversal of maladaptive remodelling of the ventricles
• Improvement in symptoms
• Improvement in prognosis.

Studies suggest that in correctly selected patients with heart failure, CRT can lead to:
• Improved functional status
• Reduced hospitalization
• Improved symptoms
• Improved quality of life
• Increased exercise capacity
• Reduced mortality.

CRT also improves echo endpoints including:
• Improved LV systolic function
• Reduced LV size and volumes
• Reduced MR
• LV 'reverse remodelling' as indicated by decreased systolic and diastolic diameters and volumes.

Uses of echo in CRT

1. Patient selection – identifying potential responders to treatment (see above)
2. Optimization of CRT following device implantation
3. Monitoring and assessing progress and outcome.

1. PATIENT SELECTION FOR CRT

Several large clinical studies have based selection of patients for CRT upon ECG criteria and some (e.g. CARE-HF and EchoCRT) have also examined whether evidence suggests a beneficial role for echo. It was considered that echo might be of help in CRT in the selection of patients and the prediction of who may respond to treatment and those who can avoid an unnecessary procedure (e.g. wide QRS non-responders). Studies suggested that about 30% of these patients are non-responders and proposed that echo assessment may be helpful by determining mechanical dyssynchrony.

Echo assessment of mechanical dyssynchrony – interventricular and LV dyssynchrony

Echo can evaluate mechanical dyssynchrony. Several techniques are used. These include M-mode, 2-D echo and Doppler techniques with TDI and newer techniques, including speckle tracking echo (STE) and 3-D echo, some of which are complex and require considerable post-processing and analysis.

TDI is extensively used. Methods include pulsed wave TDI, colour-coded TDI, tissue tracking, displacement mapping, strain and strain rate imaging, and tissue synchronization imaging (TSI).

Echo can be used to examine both interventricular (LV to RV) and LV intraventricular dyssynchrony. No one technique is ideal to predict response to CRT, and a combination should be used. LV dyssynchrony predicts response to CRT more accurately than interventricular dyssynchrony.

Other factors that may influence response to CRT include:
• Coronary venous anatomy – impacts on LV lead placement and can be assessed by venography (Fig. 4.32)
• Presence of scar tissue – affects lead placement and can be assessed by echo, MRI and nuclear medicine techniques such as technetium-99m labelling.

Echo techniques to assess mechanical dyssynchrony

M-mode
• Parasternal long-axis septal to posterior wall motion delay of over 130 ms is a marker of LV dyssynchrony.

2-D echo
• A semi-automated endocardial border detection method can be used. Echo contrast can optimize LV border detection. Apical 4-chamber views looking at the septal to lateral wall relationship can generate wall motion curves. Computer-generated regional wall motion movement curves are compared by mathematical trace analysis based on Fourier transformation to measure LV dyssynchrony. With LV border detection, regional and fractional

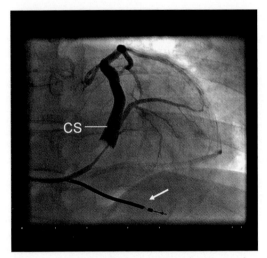

Figure 4.32 Coronary venogram prior to insertion of coronary sinus (CS) lead for CRT. The RV lead is shown (arrow).

area changes are determined and plotted versus time, yielding displacement maps. From these, LV dyssynchrony is determined. Some patients with extensive LV dyssynchrony exhibit an immediate improvement in haemodynamics with CRT.

Pulsed wave and continuous wave Doppler

- Flow across the LVOT and RVOT. With simultaneous ECG recording, it is possible to determine the delay between QRS onset and flow onset. This gives aortic and pulmonary pre-ejection periods (A-PEP and P-PEP), markers of electro-mechanical delay (EMD). Normal A-PEP is <140 ms. A-PEP increase alone as a marker of LV dyssynchrony is not a useful predictor for CRT. Interventricular mechanical delay (A-PEP minus P-PEP) is usually under 40 ms. A delay of >40 ms is a marker of interventricular dyssynchrony. This measure may be more helpful in CRT assessment.
- Transmitral pulsed wave Doppler can be used to measure diastolic filling time (time from onset of mitral E-wave to the end of the A-wave) as a percentage of the cardiac cycle length. The normal value is >40%. Alone, this is not a useful measure for predicting CRT response, but may help at baseline and CRT follow-up.

Tissue Doppler imaging (TDI) and speckle tracking echo (STE)

TDI techniques are widely used to assess dyssynchrony. STE techniques (e.g. for strain analysis) are also used. These are discussed in more detail in Section 7.9. TDI techniques include:

- **Pulsed wave TDI**, with 2-, 4- or 12-segment models of LV dyssynchrony, is used to predict response to CRT. TDI measures the velocity of longitudinal cardiac motion and allows comparison of timing of wall motion in relation to electrical activity, giving EMD. Different parameters are derived (e.g. peak systolic velocity, time to peak systolic velocity). Only one segment can be examined at a time. It is time consuming and cannot compare segments simultaneously. Measurements are influenced by heart rate, load conditions and respiration. Timing of peak systolic velocity is often difficult to identify, giving imprecise LV dyssynchrony information. This method cannot differentiate between active and passive movement of myocardial segments. TDI can also assess interventricular dyssynchrony by comparing the delay between peak systolic velocity of LV and RV free walls.

- **Colour-coded TDI** can be used to assess LV dyssynchrony. Colour-coded images need post-processing. Tracings can be used to show the time to peak systolic velocity. Initially, an apical 4-chamber view was used. Velocity tracings were derived from the basal, septal and lateral segments and septal to lateral delay was measured. A delay of >60 ms predicted acute response to CRT. Subsequently, a 4-segment model was applied, which included septal, lateral, inferior and anterior segments. A delay of >65 ms predicted response to CRT.

- **Tissue tracking.** This is calculated as the integral of the velocity curve with time and shows the displacement of tissue during the cycle. It does not distinguish between active and passive movement of a segment. It provides a colour-coded display of myocardial displacement, allowing for easy visualization of LV dyssynchrony and the region of latest activation.

- **Strain and strain rate analysis.** Strain is a dimensionless measure of myocardial deformation, which gives an assessment of myocardial mechanics (see also Sections 4.7 and 7.9). Strain is the fractional or percentage change in an object's dimension compared to its original dimension. Strain rate is the speed at which deformation occurs. These can help to distinguish active systolic contraction and passive motion of segments. This is important (e.g. in patients with ischaemic cardiomyopathy in the presence of scar tissue). Offline analysis of the colour-coded TDI images is needed. Timing of events during the cardiac cycle can be measured accurately. A disadvantage is that, with TDI, it is angle-dependent and easily influenced by noise.

- **Tissue synchronization imaging (TSI).** TSI is a signal-processing algorithm of TDI data, to detect and colour encode peak myocardial velocities. Colour-coded information can be superimposed on 2-D echo images, providing visual and mechanical information related to anatomical region. LV dyssynchrony can be shown as differences in times to peak velocity of opposing walls (e.g. inferoseptal to lateral wall [4-chamber view], anterior to inferior wall [2-chamber view] and anteroseptal to posterior wall [long-axis view]). Multi-plane TSI can give 3-D reconstruction of colour coded LV activation.

3-D echo in CRT

3-D echo can be used to:

- Assess LV volumes and LVEF.
- Examine regional wall motion abnormalities. This gives an indication of LV dyssynchrony (analysis of regional function) and the degree of dispersion of segmental volume changes. The change in volume for each segment (using 16 or 17 segment models of LV) throughout the cycle can be shown. With synchronous contraction, each segment is expected to achieve its minimum volume at almost the same point of the cardiac cycle. In LV dyssynchrony, dispersion exists in the timing of the point of minimum volume for each segment. The degree of dispersion reflects the severity of LV dyssynchrony.
- Quantify valvular regurgitation (e.g. MR).
- Guide electrophysiologists in selecting optimum lead placement positions by using parametric 'polar map' displays of the 3-D data of the timing of LV contraction.

Currently, no extensive data are available on the prediction of response to CRT using 3-D echo.

2. OPTIMIZATION OF CRT FOLLOWING DEVICE IMPLANTATION

Echo also plays a role in the optimization of pacemaker settings after CRT. Changes in atrioventricular and interventricular pacing delays can improve the benefit from CRT (Fig. 4.33). The response to CRT leads to some immediate benefits (acute improvement in haemodynamic parameters such as cardiac output and improvements in MR) and long-term benefits (improvement in clinical parameters, systolic LV function, reverse LV remodelling and further reduction in MR).

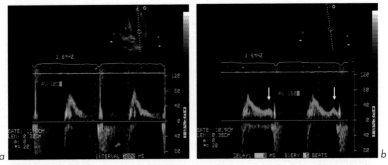

a   b

Figure 4.33 CRT optimization. Pulsed wave Doppler at LV inflow. Changing the atrioventricular time interval from **(a)** 100 ms to **(b)** 180 ms, by altering the pacemaker settings, improves LV filling with the emergence of an A-wave (arrows).

Optimization of atrioventricular and interventricular (VV) delays in CRT

Optimization of these pacemaker settings may further enhance the benefit from CRT. Both atrioventricular and VV delays can be optimized using modern CRT devices. Doppler echo can be used to optimize atrioventricular delay (Fig. 4.33). This echo-guided optimization appears crucial in some patients with heart failure, who may exhibit an acute increase in cardiac output of up to 50%. It is carried out by determining the optimum atrioventricular delay to allow the end of the Doppler A-wave, corresponding to LA contraction, to occur just before the onset of aortic systolic Doppler flow. The effects of optimization can also be examined by looking at the reduction in LV dyssynchrony and increases in LVEF.

Reduction in MR

Reduction in MR has been reported after CRT and can be improved by VV optimization. The severity of MR can be examined by echo Doppler techniques.

3. ECHO ASSESSMENT OF RESPONSE FOLLOWING CRT

Use of echo to monitor and assess long-term progress and outcome of CRT

Despite acute improvements with CRT, deciding who is a long-term responder to CRT can be difficult to assess objectively and to quantify. There is a placebo effect with CRT in about 40% of patients.

Small studies initially used invasive methods to assess acute haemodynamic response to CRT. Long-term response is usually assessed at 3–6 months of CRT. It is mainly evaluated by clinical or echo parameters. The relationship between acute haemodynamic response and chronic outcomes is still not entirely clear.

In patients who improve clinically following CRT, clinical and echo response may not occur simultaneously. Some patients who show clinical improvement may not exhibit improved echo parameters, such as reverse remodelling (which can be defined as >15% reduction in LV end-systolic volume) and vice versa. More patients exhibit improved clinical parameters than improved echo markers (Box 4.2). This discrepancy further complicates the initial selection of patients.

CRT leads to changes in LV size, LV volumes, LVEF and reverse remodelling (indicated by decreases in LV systolic and diastolic diameters and volumes, Fig. 4.34), and improves LV and interventricular dyssynchrony. Echo can help to measure these

Box 4.2 Markers of long-term response to CRT

Clinical

- New York Heart Association (NYHA) functional class
- Quality-of-life score
- 6-minute walk distance
- Peak VO_2 exercise capacity
- Heart failure hospitalizations
- Cardiac mortality

Echo

- LVEF
- LV dimensions/volumes
- Reverse remodelling
- MR
- Interventricular resynchronization
- LV resynchronization

Adapted from Bax JJ, Abraham T, Barold SS, et al. Cardiac resynchronization therapy: part 2 – issues during and after device implantation and unresolved questions. J Am Coll Cardiol. 2005;46:2168–2182.

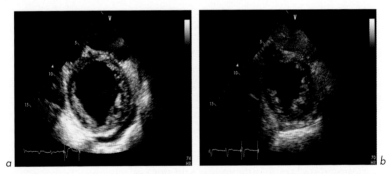

a   *b*

Figure 4.34 Reverse remodelling following CRT. Parasternal short-axis views showing LV at end-diastole at **(a)** baseline and **(b)** 6 months following implantation of CRT device. LV end-diastolic volume has decreased.

changes. The ultimate clinical endpoints include a reduction in hospitalization and mortality rates.

Guidelines

Guidelines have been prepared suggesting which patients with heart failure may benefit from CRT (see Box 4.3). These may change as further clinical information becomes available.

Box 4.3 Indications for ICDs and CRT for arrhythmias and heart failure (based upon NICE technology appraisal guidance [TA314] June 2014)

ICDs are recommended as options for:

• Treating people with previous serious ventricular arrhythmia who, without a treatable cause:
  • have survived a cardiac arrest due to VT or VF **or**
  • have spontaneous sustained VT causing syncope or haemodynamic compromise **or**
  • have sustained VT without syncope or cardiac arrest and also have LVEF ≤ 35% but heart failure symptoms are no worse than NYHA class III
• Treating people who:
  • have a familial cardiac condition with a high risk of sudden death, e.g. long QT syndrome, HCM, Brugada syndrome or arrhythmogenic cardiomyopathy **or**
  • have undergone surgical repair of congenital heart disease

ICDs, CRT with defibrillator (CRT-D) or CRT with pacing (CRT-P) are recommended as options for people with heart failure who have LV dysfunction with LVEF ≤ 35%, according to NYHA class, QRS duration and presence of LBBB:

QRS interval	NYHA class I	NYHA class II	NYHA class III	NYHA class IV
<120 milliseconds	ICD if there is a high risk of sudden cardiac death			ICD and CRT not clinically indicated
120–149 milliseconds without LBBB	ICD	ICD	ICD	CRT-P
120–149 milliseconds with LBBB	ICD	CRT-D	CRT-P or CRT-D	CRT-P
≥150 milliseconds with or without LBBB	CRT-D	CRT-D	CRT-P or CRT-D	CRT-P

TRANSOESOPHAGEAL, 3-D AND STRESS ECHO AND OTHER ECHO TECHNIQUES

5.1 TRANSOESOPHAGEAL ECHO

The echo techniques described so far have used ultrasound directed from the chest wall – transthoracic echo (TTE). The oesophagus in its mid-course lies posterior to and very close to the heart and ascending aorta and anterior to the descending aorta (Fig. 5.1).

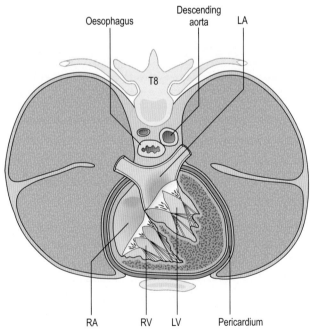

Figure 5.1 Cross-section of thorax at the 8th thoracic vertebra level (from above).

An echo technique exists for examining the heart with a transducer in the oesophagus – transoesophageal echo (TOE) (Figs. 5.2, 5.3, 5.4, 5.5). In some countries, the abbreviation used is TEE. This uses a transducer mounted upon a modified probe similar to those used for upper gastrointestinal endoscopy and allows examination of the heart without the barrier to ultrasound usually provided by the ribs, chest wall and lungs. By advancing the probe tip to various depths in the oesophagus and stomach, manoeuvring the tip of the transducer and by altering the angle of the ultrasound beam with controls placed on the handle, several different views of the heart can be obtained.

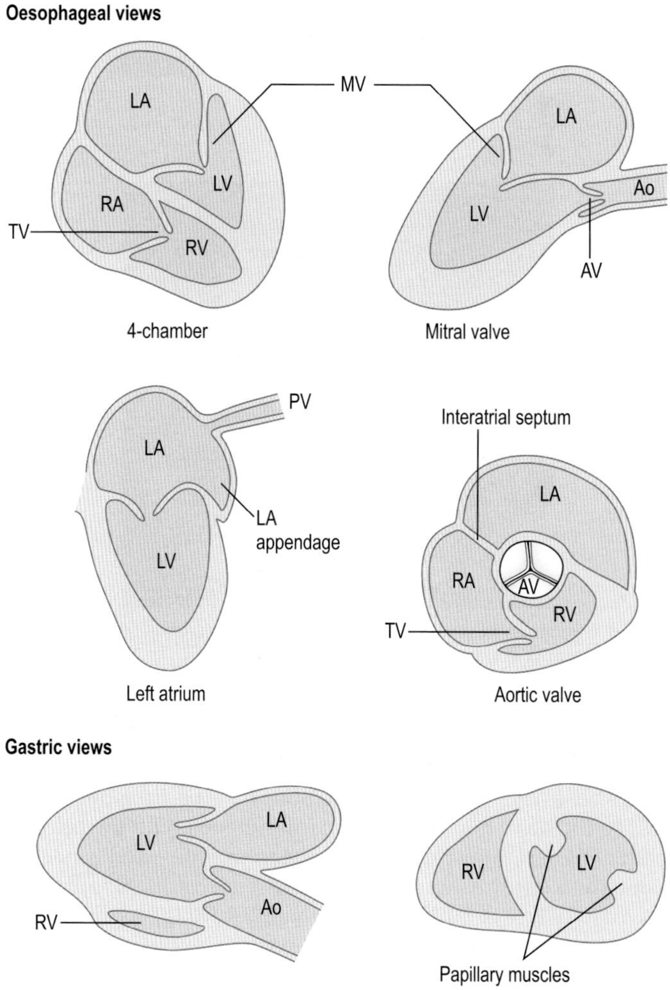

Oesophageal views

Gastric views

Figure 5.2 Standard TOE views.

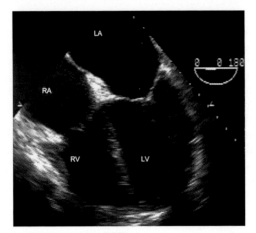

Figure 5.3 4-chamber view using TOE.

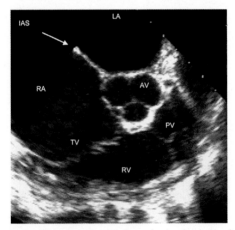

Figure 5.4 Structures at aortic valve level on short-axis view using TOE. The interatrial septum is shown (arrow).

ADVANTAGES OF TOE

- Improved image quality and resolution – the transducer is very close to the heart and there is less interference with the ultrasound beam. Higher ultrasound frequencies can be used since tissue attenuation of ultrasound is small and penetration depth required less than TTE (e.g. 5 MHz rather than 2–4 MHz).
- Some aspects of the heart can be examined that cannot be seen clearly using TTE, e.g. posterior parts such as LA appendage, descending aorta and pulmonary veins.

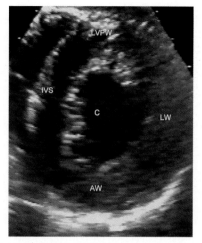

Figure 5.5 Short-axis view of left ventricle using TOE – transgastric view. *AW,* anterior wall; *C,* cavity; *IVS,* interventricular septum; *LVPW,* left ventricular posterior wall; *LW,* lateral wall.

DISADVANTAGES OF TOE

* Invasive technique – uncomfortable with potential small risk
* New views have to be learnt.

Because of the invasive nature of TOE, it should only be performed if there is a good indication and after TTE has been performed. TOE-derived information should be used to complement that derived from TTE and not as an alternative. The potential risks of TOE (e.g. oesophageal damage) should be weighed up carefully against the potential benefits.

USES OF TOE

* **Mitral valve disease** – stenosis (anatomy of valve and subvalvular apparatus and assessment of suitability for valve repair rather than replacement or for balloon mitral valvotomy); prolapse (suitability for repair); regurgitation (severity and suitability for repair) (Fig. 5.6)
* **Endocarditis** – vegetations; abscess
* **Prosthetic valves** – haemodynamics; stability; endocarditis
* **Aortic disease** – dissection of ascending, arch or descending thoracic aorta; trauma; atheroma
* **Aortic valve disease**
* **Thromboembolic vascular disease** – stroke/TIA or peripheral embolism
* **Left atrial appendage** – thrombus
* **Intracardiac masses** – myxoma or other tumour; thrombus

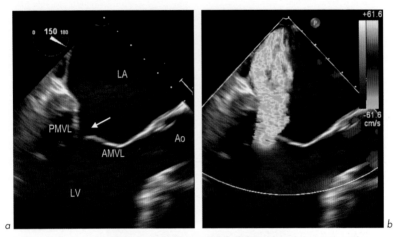

Figure 5.6 Severe mitral regurgitation on TOE. **(a)** Failure of coaptation of anterior and posterior mitral valve leaflets, due to restriction of posterior mitral valve leaflet. A defect is shown (arrow). **(b)** Severe mitral regurgitation on colour flow Doppler. TOE mitral valve view.

- **Septal defects** – Atrial (especially assessment for suitability for percutaneous closure); ventricular; contrast studies
- **Intraoperative monitoring** – assessment of MV repair; LV function and regional wall motion abnormalities; myomectomy
- **Congenital heart disease** – anatomy; haemodynamic assessment
- **Critically ill people in ICU**
- **Air or fat embolism** – haemodynamics.

PATIENT PREPARATION AND CARE DURING TOE

The patient should give informed consent being aware of the potential risks, which include:
- Oesophageal trauma or perforation
- The risks of intravenous sedation
- Aspiration of stomach contents into lungs.

The patient should have fasted for at least 4 hours. All false and loose teeth should be removed. There should be no history of difficulty in swallowing solids or liquids (dysphagia), which might suggest oesophageal disease. It is advisable to give oxygen during the procedure via nasal cannulae, to monitor blood oxygen with a pulse oximeter and to have suction equipment available to remove saliva from the mouth. Continuous ECG monitoring should be carried out as with any echo examination. Resuscitation equipment should be available.

A local anaesthetic spray (e.g. lidocaine [lignocaine] 10%) is used on the pharynx. Several sprays are given and there may be some systemic absorption. Intravenous sedation with a short-acting agent such as the benzodiazepine, midazolam, is often used. The patient is placed in the left lateral position with the neck fully flexed to aid insertion of the transducer into the oesophagus. A plastic bite guard is placed in the mouth to protect the transducer and the fingers of the person performing the TOE.

It is unusual to need to give a general anaesthetic (e.g. if TOE is considered essential and the patient is unable to tolerate the procedure under local anaesthesia and intravenous sedation). TOE is often carried out as a day-case procedure. After the procedure, the patient should not eat or drink for at least 1 hour (to prevent aspiration into the lungs or burning of the throat) since the throat remains numb and the patient may still be drowsy.

CONTRAINDICATIONS TO TOE

- Inability or refusal of the patient to give informed consent
- Dysphagia of unknown cause
- Oesophageal disease – tumour, oesophagitis, oesophageal varices, diverticulum, stricture, Mallory–Weiss tear, tracheo-oesophageal fistula
- Severe cervical arthritis or instability
- Bleeding gastric ulcer
- Severe pulmonary disease with hypoxaemia.

COMPLICATIONS OF TOE (0.2–0.5%)

- Trauma – ranges from minor bleeding to oesophageal perforation
- Hypoxia
- Arrhythmia – SVT, AF, VT
- Laryngospasm or bronchospasm
- Angina
- Drug-related – respiratory depression, allergic reaction.

SPECIFIC USES OF TOE

1. Cardiac or aortic source of embolism

TOE is often carried out in young patients (aged <50 years) who have had a stroke. Approximately 20% may have a cardiac embolic source.

Detection of intracardiac thrombus with TTE is difficult with a high false-negative rate despite high suspicion on clinical grounds. TOE is superior not only because of improved image resolution but also because it is better at viewing areas where thrombus is likely to occur, such as LA appendage (Fig. 5.7, and see Fig. 6.3). This is the most common site for thrombus, usually in patients with underlying heart disease.

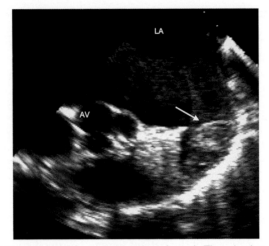

Figure 5.7 Thrombus in left atrial appendage (arrow). There is also spontaneous echo contrast in the left atrial cavity.

Risk factors for LA thrombus include:
- MV disease (especially MS)
- AF
- LA dilatation
- Low-output states (e.g. heart failure).

In some studies of patients with cerebral ischaemia (TIA and stroke), up to 5% had LA thrombus and in 75% of cases this was in the LA appendage. Thrombus may appear as a rounded or ovoid mass that may completely fill the appendage. False-positive diagnosis of thrombus may occur due to misinterpretation of LA anatomy:

1. Trabeculation of LA may be misdiagnosed as small thrombi

2. The ridge between the LA appendage and left upper pulmonary vein may be misdiagnosed as thrombus.

Spontaneous echo contrast
A swirling 'smoke-like' pattern of echo densities within any cardiac chamber is known as spontaneous contrast (Fig. 5.7). It is usually seen in low-output states. It is most often seen in the LA in mitral disease (up to one-third of cases), especially MS where it may occur in up to 50% of cases. It is due to sluggish flow and is associated with clumping of red cells (rouleaux formation), which become more echo-reflective. There is an increased thromboembolic risk – LA thrombus occurs in 20–30% of those with spontaneous contrast.

Other LA structural abnormalities associated with increased thromboembolic risk include ASD, patent foramen ovale (PFO) and atrial septal aneurysm.

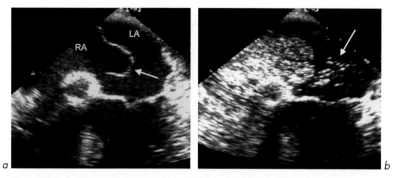

Figure 5.8 Atrial septal aneurysm on TOE study. **(a)** Aneurysm bulging into left atrium (arrow). There appears to be a defect at lower region of aneurysm, probably a patent foramen ovale (PFO). **(b)** Bubble contrast study showing bubbles crossing from right atrium to left atrium (arrow) through an associated PFO.

Atrial septal aneurysm

This is a bulging of the fossa ovalis and is found at autopsy in 1% of people (Fig. 5.8). For echo purposes, the bulge must involve 1.5 cm of the septum and protrude 1.1 cm into either atrium. It is found in 0.2% of TTE series. In suspected cardiac source of embolism, it occurs in up to 15% of cases. The association with TIA/stroke may be because the aneurysm is thrombogenic and/or due to its frequent association with PFO and ASDs, which may allow paradoxical right-to-left embolization. TOE can help to detect all of these. A bubble contrast study during TOE can help to identify a small ASD or PFO and show a small shunt (Section 6.4).

TOE can show thrombus in other parts of the heart (e.g. LV mural thrombus). This is detected in over 40% of cases of acute MI at autopsy. Usually this occurs in the presence of anterior infarction and apical dyskinesis or LV aneurysm. Thrombus can also form in other low-output states, especially with chamber enlargement or where there is foreign material in the heart (e.g. pacing leads, central lines, prosthetic valves), particularly if inadequately anticoagulated or malfunctioning.

2. Examination of the aorta (see Section 6.5)

TTE only gives good images of the ascending aorta, aortic arch and proximal descending aorta in a small minority of adults. TOE can add to this by providing excellent imaging of the aortic root, proximal ascending aorta, distal aortic arch and descending thoracic aorta. The interposition of the trachea between the oesophagus and ascending aorta limits the ability to image the upper ascending aorta and proximal aortic arch.

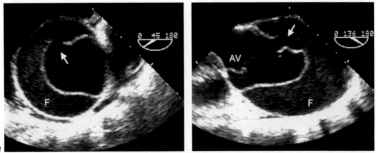

a   b

Figure 5.9 Dissecting aneurysm of the aortic root and ascending aorta – TOE. **(a)** Short-axis view and **(b)** long-axis view of the ascending aorta showing dissection intimal flap with entry point (arrow). There is spontaneous contrast in the false lumen (F).

Aortic dimensions and dilatation

TOE allows accurate determination of aortic dimensions and reveals dilatation seen in aortic aneurysm (Fig. 6.25).

Aortic atheroma

TOE helps detect and differentiate mobile and immobile atheromatous plaques. Mobile plaques may be associated with a higher embolic rate, as are pedunculated rather than linear plaques. Atheromatous plaques in the ascending aorta are found by TOE in at least 1% of people who have experienced an embolic CVA.

Aortic dissection

TOE is the best technique for the diagnosis of aortic dissection, particularly of the ascending aorta where surgical intervention is urgent (Figs. 5.9, 6.26, 7.2). TOE makes the diagnosis with sensitivity and specificity around 98%, better than angiography or CT scanning. Dissection of the descending thoracic aorta can also be identified.

3. Endocarditis

TTE should always be used in the initial assessment of suspected or definite endocarditis. The superior spatial resolution provided by TOE allows small vegetations of only 1–2 mm to be identified and their location and morphology to be examined (Figs. 6.4, 6.8). All valves can be examined, but TOE is especially useful for the mitral and aortic valves (right-sided vegetations are often large and can be detected by TTE). In aortic subacute bacterial endocarditis (SBE), TOE is especially useful for aortic root abscess (TOE shows over 85% of such cases, TTE less than 30%), fistula or aneurysm of the sinus of Valsalva.

TOE is of use in endocarditis:
• Where TTE has not been diagnostic
• To assess the size, location and morphology of vegetations

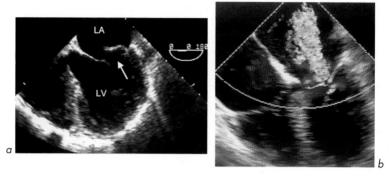

Figure 5.10 TOE showing **(a)** severe prolapse of posterior mitral valve leaflet (arrow) and **(b)** severe mitral regurgitation.

- To assess possible complications such as aortic root abscess
- In suspected infection of prosthetic valves (Fig. 6.8).

TOE should be considered in the majority of cases of suspected endocarditis.

4. Native valve assessment

Mitral valve

TTE is good but some aspects may be difficult to assess. The posterior leaflet may be poorly visualized, especially if calcified or in the presence of mitral annular calcification. TOE can provide essential information in planning intervention such as MV repair (Figs. 5.6, 5.10, 5.11).

In MR, quantitative assessment of severity by TTE is difficult. TOE allows a more thorough assessment by Doppler and colour flow of the degree of MR within the LA. Severity can also be assessed by the pattern of pulmonary venous flow (severe MR may be associated with reversal of flow). The morphology of the valve can be examined to assess if suitable for valve repair rather than replacement. The exact segment of the valve that is causing regurgitation can be identified.

TOE can be used intraoperatively to assess the adequacy of valve repair.

In MS, TOE is very useful in deciding if a stenosed MV is suitable for balloon valvuloplasty or whether surgical treatment such as mitral valvotomy or replacement is needed.

Balloon valvuloplasty for MS is **not** suitable if:

- The anterior MV leaflet is immobile, thickened or calcified
- The chordae are thickened or calcified
- The leaflet tips are heavily calcified
- There is more than mild MR
- There is visible thrombus (e.g. in LA appendage).

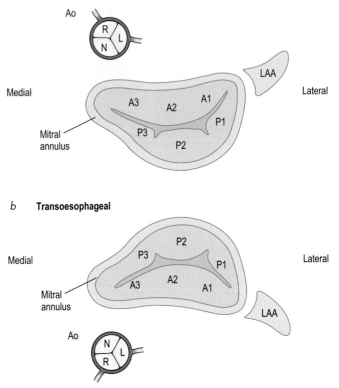

Figure 5.11 Mitral valve viewed from **(a)** transthoracic parasternal view and **(b)** transoesophageal mid-gastric view. The 3 scallops of the anterior (A1, A2, A3) and posterior (P1, P2, P3) leaflets, the left atrial appendage (LAA) and the position of the proximal aorta (Ao) are shown. *N*, non-coronary sinus; *R*, right coronary sinus; *L*, left coronary sinus.

Aortic valve

TOE allows confident prediction of the integrity and number of cusps, evaluation of the aortic root, aortic sinuses and LVOT. Morphological assessment of AV can help give an indication of the aetiology of AR and colour flow mapping gives an indication of severity.

TOE is useful in preparation and during the newer AV intervention procedures, such as TAVI and TAVR (Section 6.5).

Tricuspid and pulmonary valves and right heart

The TV does not lend itself particularly well to TOE. Views can be obtained, but TTE is often sufficient. The PV, right ventricular outflow tract (RVOT) and proximal pulmonary artery can also be imaged reasonably well by TOE. It is often possible to view the 4 pulmonary veins and their connections with the LA, or to determine if there is partial or total anomalous pulmonary venous drainage.

5. Prosthetic valve assessment (see Section 6.3)

This is one of the most important indications for TOE. The close proximity of the transducer to the valve, the reduction in interfering tissues nearby and enhanced spatial resolution make this very useful and superior to TTE.

The MV position is particularly well examined because of the orientation relative to the transducer. Paravalvular MR is well detected and may occur in up to 2.5% of all MV prostheses (Fig. 6.7). TOE can be used intraoperatively and post-operatively to assess the presence and severity of paraprosthetic MR. TOE is useful in distinguishing between mild, moderate and severe paraprosthetic MR (the latter may deteriorate progressively and require re-operation). Vegetations due to infection on prosthetic valves can be detected (Fig. 6.8). Shadowing of the LVOT occurs with mitral prostheses and may limit the ability to detect AR.

For aortic prostheses, TOE also has advantages over TTE, especially in biological valve degeneration, obstruction of prosthesis, regurgitation, abscesses or mass lesions (vegetations, thrombus). There are still some limitations even with TOE. The imaging planes are limited and as a result the acoustic shadow generated by mechanical prostheses may hide lesions in some areas. Aortic prostheses leave a portion of the aortic annulus immune from interrogation, which may lead to underdiagnosis of root abscess.

6. Congenital disease (see Section 6.4)

TOE plays an important role, especially in paediatric practice and in complex congenital heart disease. It may help diagnose and assess severity and haemodynamics in:
- Intracardiac shunts – PFO (Fig. 6.14), ASD (Figs. 5.12, 6.12, 6.13), VSD (Figs. 6.9, 6.10)
- Extracardiac shunt – patent ductus arteriosus (PDA)
- Congenital valvular abnormalities
- Aortic coarctation
- Anomalous systemic or pulmonary venous connections
- Follow-up of corrective or palliative procedures.

7. Cardiac and paracardiac masses (see Section 6.1)

TOE is superior to TTE in a number of settings and should be considered if TTE does not adequately visualize masses, particularly in:
- LA and appendage (Figs. 5.7, 6.3)
- Descending thoracic aorta

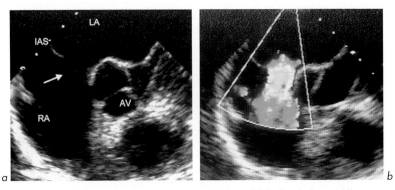

a | b

Figure 5.12 Ostium secundum atrial septal defect. **(a)** Defect in interatrial septum (IAS) measuring 16 mm shown at TOE examination (arrow). **(b)** Colour flow mapping showing flow from left to right atrium.

- Pericardium
- PA
- Right-sided paracardiac region
- SVC and IVC
- Anterior mediastinum.

5.2 STRESS ECHO

Stress transthoracic echo aids in the diagnosis of ischaemic heart disease. It helps to localize the site and quantifies the extent of ischaemia by the demonstration of regional wall motion and thickness abnormalities with stress that are not present at rest (Figs. 5.13 and 5.14). This technique may be used as an alternative to exercise stress ECG testing or stress radionuclide myocardial perfusion scanning (e.g. stress thallium) in certain circumstances. Stress may be by:

- Physical exercise (treadmill or bicycle)
- Pharmacological means (by the continuous infusion of an agent such as the vasodilating inotropic agent, dobutamine, or vasodilators that divert blood from areas served by stenosed arteries to other regions, e.g. dipyridamole or adenosine)
- Temporary cardiac pacing (used to increase heart rate, but invasive).

The sensitivity of stress echo is around 80% and the specificity around 90%. These compare favourably with exercise ECG testing, which has a sensitivity of around 70% and a specificity of around 80%.

Stress echo is also used in some centres to determine the extent of LVOTO associated with HCM when septal ablation by catheter instillation of ethanol or surgical myomectomy are being considered. A resting LVOT gradient of 30 mmHg in these cases may increase to over 100 mmHg during stress and may indicate the need for septal reduction.

INDICATIONS FOR STRESS ECHO

Ischaemic heart disease (Figs. 5.13, 5.14)

1. Uncertain diagnosis, equivocal exercise stress ECG test
2. Inability to exercise on treadmill
3. Resting ECG abnormality prevents interpretation of changes with exercise (e.g. LBBB, LVH with strain, digoxin)
4. Following acute MI
5. Localization of site of ischaemia
6. Assessment of myocardial viability – hibernation or stunning
7. Evaluation following revascularization (e.g. PCI ± stent or CABG)
8. Stress echo is especially useful in the assessment of possible ischaemic heart disease:
   - In women with chest pain and cardiovascular risk factors
   - Following heart transplantation
   - Prior to renal transplantation
   - Prior to vascular surgery.

LVOTO

1. HCM – to assess the LVOTO gradient with stress when considering septal ablation or resection
2. Upper septal bulge. Seen in elderly people due to fibrosis and hypertrophy. Unusually causes LVOTO.

Assessment of changes in cardiac haemodynamics with stress

1. Valve area and pressure difference (e.g. AV area in calcific AS)
2. Severity of valvular regurgitation (e.g. MR)
3. PASP (e.g. in MS or MR)
4. Pressure difference across stenosis in aortic coarctation
5. HCM to assess LVOTO.

LIMITATIONS OF STRESS ECHO

- Failure to achieve adequate workload
- Poor endocardial definition – helped by contrast echo techniques
- Complications of procedure.

COMPLICATIONS OF STRESS ECHO

This is a safe procedure if carried out with care. The rate of major complications is <0.5%.

- Major – sustained VT, sustained SVT, myocardial infarction, hypotension
- Minor – flushing, dizziness, dyspnoea, ectopic beats or non-sustained SVT, anticholinergic side effects with atropine.

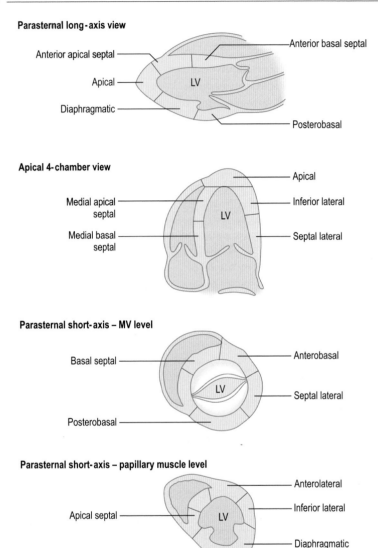

Parasternal long-axis view

Anterior apical septal

Apical

Diaphragmatic

Anterior basal septal

LV

Posterobasal

Apical 4-chamber view

Medial apical septal

Medial basal septal

Apical

Inferior lateral

LV

Septal lateral

Parasternal short-axis – MV level

Basal septal

Posterobasal

Anterobasal

LV

Septal lateral

Parasternal short-axis – papillary muscle level

Apical septal

Anterolateral

Inferior lateral

LV

Diaphragmatic

Figure 5.13 16-segment model of left ventricular myocardium. This model is appropriate for studies assessing wall motion, as the tip of the apex does not move. Adapted from Schiller NB, Shah PM, Crawford M, et al. Recommendations for quantitation of the left ventricle by two-dimensional echocardiography. American Society of Echocardiography Committee on Standards, Subcommittee on Quantitation of Two-Dimensional Echocardiograms. *J Am Soc Echocardiogr.* 1989;2:358–367.

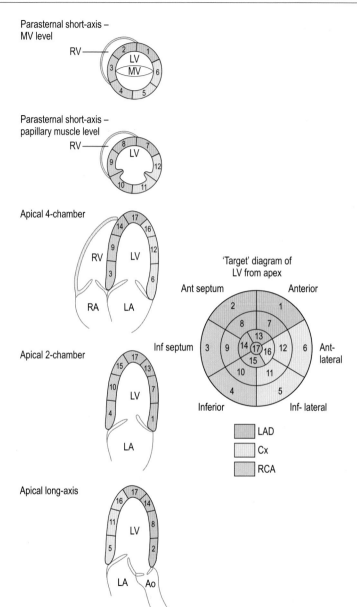

Parasternal short-axis – MV level

Parasternal short-axis – papillary muscle level

Apical 4-chamber

Apical 2-chamber

Apical long-axis

'Target' diagram of LV from apex

Figure 5.14 17-segment model of left ventricular myocardium. Differs from 16-segment model by addition of apical cap (segment 17), imaging of which has improved with contrast and harmonic echo. Used predominantly for myocardial perfusion studies or to compare with other imaging modalities (e.g. cardiac CT or MRI). Arterial territories are shown: *LAD*, left anterior descending; *Cx*, circumflex; *RCA*, right coronary artery. Adapted from Cerueira MD, Weissman NJ, Dilsizian V, et al. Standardized myocardial segmentation and nomenclature for tomographic imaging of the heart. A statement for healthcare professionals from the Cardiac Imaging Committee of the Council on Clinical Cardiology of the American Heart Association. *Circulation.* 2002;105:539–542.

5.3 CONTRAST ECHO

Contrast agents can be injected into the bloodstream resulting in increased echogenicity of the blood or myocardium. This can produce opacification of the cardiac chambers or an increase in echogenicity of the myocardium. Ultrasound 'contrast' is generated by the presence of microbubbles. At low ultrasound power outputs, microbubbles scatter ultrasound at the gas–liquid interface, resulting in detection of a reflected signal by the transducer. In addition, ultrasound causes compression and expansion (i.e. oscillation), of microbubbles. The resonant frequency of a microbubble is related to its diameter. Harmonic imaging can detect this non-linear resonant signal. At high power outputs, ultrasound results in microbubble destruction. Careful adjustment of instrument power output is needed during contrast echo.

Echo contrast agents

There are 2 types of echo contrast agent:
1. Those that opacify the right heart
2. Those that opacify the left heart and myocardium.

When the size of the microbubbles is greater than the pulmonary capillary diameter, they are trapped in the capillaries and no contrast enters the left side of the heart in the absence of an intracardiac right to left communication. Left heart and myocardial contrast is achieved using microbubbles in the 1–5 μm range, which cross the pulmonary capillary bed. Microbubbles in this size range resonate with a frequency of 1.5–7 MHz, corresponding to clinical transducer frequencies.

Right heart contrast

The most widely used contrast for right heart studies is agitated saline. A simple approach is rapidly to push 5 mL of sterile saline with a small amount (approximately 0.1 mL) of air or the patient's blood between 2 syringes connecting with 3-way stop-cock taps. This results in the production of large diameter microbubbles that do not pass through the pulmonary capillary bed. When the saline appears opaque, it is injected rapidly into a peripheral vein during echo imaging. Care must be taken to ensure there is no visible free air in the injection system. Agitated saline should not be used in patients with known significant right-to-left shunting to avoid the risk of paradoxical embolization into the systemic circulation.

Left heart and myocardial contrast

Left heart and myocardial contrast agents consist of air or low-solubility fluorocarbon gas in stabilized microbubbles encapsulated with agents such as denatured albumin or monosaccharides. These contrasts are usually prepared just before use. Some require re-suspension before intravenous injection whilst others are diluted and given as a continuous infusion. Microbubbles are fragile, so careful handling and infusion techniques are needed. The optimum volume and infusion rate depend on the specific contrast agent used, to provide full opacification whilst minimizing attenuation due to excess microbubble density.

Applications of contrast echo

The main clinical applications of contrast echo studies are:
1. Detection of intracardiac shunt
2. LV opacification
3. Myocardial perfusion
4. Enhancement of Doppler signals.

1. Detection of intracardiac shunt. Right heart contrast allows the detection of a right-to-left intracardiac shunt. With a patent foramen ovale (PFO), shunting may be seen only after a Valsalva manoeuvre because of the transient increase in RA compared to LA pressure (Fig. 6.14). Even with a predominant left-to-right shunt (e.g. with an ASD), there is usually a small amount of right-to-left shunting when the pressures on both sides equalize, allowing detection of the shunt with right heart contrast. Right heart contrast may also be used to identify a left-sided SVC or to demonstrate the systemic venous inflow pathway in complex congenital heart disease.

2. LV opacification. In patients with poor image quality on resting studies or during stress echo, contrast enhances the identification of wall motion abnormalities and overall LV systolic function. Endocardial border detection can be enhanced (e.g. for examination of LV dyssynchrony for CRT assessment). Most centres now routinely perform contrast enhancement during stress studies when endocardial definition is suboptimal.

3. Myocardial perfusion. Myocardial perfusion with contrast echo is technically challenging. Only approximately 6% of LV stroke volume perfuses the myocardium via the coronary arteries, so the relative number of microbubbles in the coronary circulation reaching the myocardium is small. Mechanical and ultrasound destruction of microbubbles further limits contrast echo. This can be used to assess myocardial perfusion, viability and function in acute MI or during bypass surgery and during stress echo. Contrast can be injected directly into a coronary artery in certain situations (Fig. 5.15). Myocardial perfusion by echo contrast has not yet become a routine clinical test.

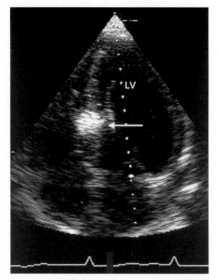

Figure 5.15 Contrast echo study in a patient with hypertrophic cardiomyopathy. Contrast has been selectively injected into the first septal branch of the left anterior descending coronary artery during cardiac catheterization and can be seen in the septum (arrow) on apical 4-chamber echo. This shows the area of myocardium that is infarcted by the technique of selective instillation of ethanol ('septal reduction').

4. Enhancement of Doppler signals. Contrast may be used to increase Doppler signal strength (e.g. a TR jet to estimate PASP). The effect of contrast on the Doppler signal varies with instruments and this approach has not gained widespread use.

Limitations of contrast echo

- Right heart contrast to detect large intracardiac shunts is infrequently needed, given the sensitivity of colour Doppler and TOE. The primary use of right heart contrast is for detection of a PFO. A small VSD usually will not be detected with right heart contrast injection because there is little right-to-left shunting.
- The use of left heart contrast requires considerable experience to judge the infusion rate and volume needed to opacify the LV optimally. When the microbubble density is too high, an excessive contrast effect at the apex results in attenuation of signal or shadowing of the rest of the LV. A swirling appearance may be seen with too little contrast or in low flow states. Bubble destruction may result in a swirling pattern with inadequate ventricular opacification.
- The addition of contrast injection to the echo examination increases the cost, duration and risk of the procedure.

- Contrast during a standard echo or stress echo study may make this approach impractical in many laboratories due to the time and personnel needed.
- Adverse reactions to contrast agents may occur, such as nausea, vomiting, headaches, flushing and dizziness. Major reactions such as hypersensitivity or anaphylaxis are rare.

5.4 THREE-DIMENSIONAL (3-D) ECHO

Advances in echo technology now allow the generation of 3-D echo images. This refers to several approaches for the acquisition and display of ultrasound images. Unlike 2-D echo (which uses a thin, single-plane beam), 3-D echo uses transducers densely packed with piezoelectric crystals to produce many scan lines giving a pyramid of ultrasound. 3-D echo allows the heart to be seen in new ways showing complex and anatomical features not possible with standard 2-D echo. Cardiac structures can be rotated or viewed from different orientations even after image acquisition. This ability to view anatomy from different viewpoints is an advantage.

3-D ultrasound is not a new concept and has been known as a clinical application in non-cardiac applications such as obstetrics for over 15 years. To be clinically useful, cardiac imaging requires high time resolution to keep up with heart movement. Previously 3-D echo involved reconstruction from multiple 2-D images. New triggering technology and high frame rate processing have allowed the development of live (real-time) 3-D echo. It is likely that much of echo will become fully 3-D in the future, but the optimum 3-D approach is evolving.

Live (real-time) 3-D echo techniques are now available that allow transthoracic and TOE studies. In some centres, these are used before and during cardiac surgery and non-surgical cardiac interventions (e.g. TAVI, Section 6.5).

With improved technical issues, live 3-D echo can impact upon patient care and improve pre-surgical planning. It is also a valuable method of communicating information to surgeons, physicians and patients. 3-D echo is particularly helpful for evaluation of valvular abnormalities such as before and during MV repair or percutaneous mitral balloon valvuloplasty and congenital heart disease. 3-D echo is being used increasingly in clinical practice. It has several clinical applications, including:
- Enhanced diagnostic capability reducing or eliminating the need for expensive or invasive tests and procedures
- Better visualization of the heart to improve surgical planning and provide intraoperative information
- Information about cardiac haemodynamics (e.g. LV function)
- Live assessments of heart valve function

- Examination of complex congenital heart abnormalities
- Teaching and research.

The basic approaches to displaying 3-D echo data are:
- Live (real-time) 3-D display
- Simultaneous 2-D image planes
- Border reconstructions.

The most intuitive is a 3-D image that can be rotated and viewed from multiple angles in real-time (see Box 5.1). Current display formats suffer from showing 3-D images on 2-D displays. This limitation should be resolved as 3-D display systems become more widely available. 3-D echo can also be used to generate multiple 2-D

Box 5.1 Live (real-time) 3-D echo allows visualization of complex cardiac anatomy and can provide:

- Assessment of regional/global function (e.g. LV function)
- Assessment of valvular function (e.g. MV, prosthetic valves)
- Visualization of complex anatomical features (e.g. congenital)
- Catheter visualization in 3-D space (e.g. during TAVI or EPS)
- Better visualization of short axis views, from apex to base of LV and RV
- Visualization of anatomy outside of the scan plane of standard 2-D views.

Techniques/modes
- **Live 3-D** – Single, thin pyramidal volume, about 50–60° × 30° – high frame rate and live imaging of structures
- **Live 3-D zoom** – User-defined volume of interest, about 30° × 30°, e.g. to assess MV
- **Live 3-D full volume** – Needs ECG gating and combines multiple pyramidal volumes to produce large 3-D volume, e.g. to assess LV size and function
- **Live 3-D colour** – With live 3-D zoom and full volume modes. Can display small jets, e.g. to quantify MR, paraprosthetic valve leaks
- **Live 3-D stress** – For use during stress echo, e.g. to assess LV regional wall motion abnormalities due to myocardial ischaemia
- **X-plane** – Not true 3-D (two 2-D images displayed side by side). Real-time imaging in 2 orthogonal planes. Excellent frame rates, e.g. to analyze anatomical structures and pathology.

image planes. As with 2-D echo, quantification from 3-D echo requires the tracing of cardiac borders. This can provide very accurate LV volume measurements and can allow detailed assessments of wall motion, myocardial thickening and LV shape. Border tracing is time-consuming and as automated edge detection programs improve, analysis time will decrease and this will become more widely used clinically.

Clinical applications of 3-D echo

1. Chamber quantification

• Quantification of ventricular volumes and function. Measurements of volume throughout the cardiac cycle, LV mass and dimensions of LV and RV. Analysis of global and regional wall motion. 3-D echo is superior to 2-D echo for both LV and RV volumes. The technique requires acquisition of 3-D echo data and manual endocardial border tracing. Since the process of tracing is time-consuming, semi-automated techniques and detection algorithms are being developed. The advent of real-time volumetric scanning will enhance the use of 3-D echo in volume measurement.

• Infarct size estimation.

• Evaluation of distorted ventricles.

• Serial LV volume measurements in individuals with valvular regurgitation to help time surgery (e.g. AR, MR).

• Assessment of RV function. This is limited by 2-D echo because of anatomical considerations including the asymmetrical pyramidal shape of RV, which does not conform to simple geometrical assumptions.

• Assessment of ventricular function in congenital cardiac lesions such as ASD and VSD.

• May be useful in assessment of patients with heart failure for CRT.

• LA volume measurement.

2. Valvular heart disease

• Real-time 3-D echo obviates many of the practical limitations in reconstructive 3-D techniques and also provides greater clinical applications in valvular heart disease, both in diagnostic evaluation and in real-time guidance during surgical valve repair.

• 3-D echo is ideally suited for assessing valve function given the non-planar anatomy of the cardiac valves and the complex anatomical changes seen in valvular heart disease.

• MV is particularly suited because of the complex relationship between the valve leaflets, subvalvular apparatus and myocardial wall. 3-D echo can give insights into MV structure and assessment of MV prolapse, endocarditis and congenital MV abnormalities. Important functional and anatomical information can be gained in

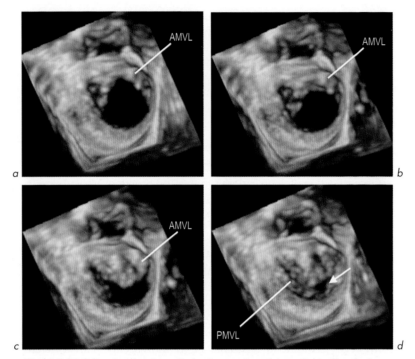

Figure 5.16 3-D echo showing mitral valve anatomy in a patient with mitral regurgitation. **(a)–(c)** Open MV at various stages of closure, showing movement of anterior MV leaflet (AMVL). **(d)** Coaptation defect (arrow) due to restriction of P2 segment of posterior MV leaflet (PMVL). The MV is viewed from the perspective of the left atrium.

ischaemic and functional MR resulting from derangement of the normal relationship between MV leaflets, annulus and LV. The technique is useful in guiding surgical repair of the MV. Real-time 3-D images can be rotated and cropped at different levels to show different views. For example, the MV can be viewed from the perspective of the LA (Fig. 5.16). This is helpful for surgeons during MV repair. Real-time 3-D is useful in quantifying MR and reconstruction of jets. It can be used for assessment of MS (Fig. 5.17) and calculation of MV area. 3-D echo has been used for guidance of percutaneous mitral valvuloplasty.

- AV. 3-D echo has been applied for anatomical assessment of AV and root morphology and to calculate valve area. It shows aortic flow patterns and quantifies AR. AV vegetations can be localized. Congenital outflow obstruction can be demonstrated, as can outflow changes in AV after balloon dilatation. AV can be viewed from the perspective of the aorta and from a transgastric view.

- TV and PV. 3-D echo has been used to show abnormalities in rheumatic and degenerative TV and PV disease and allows

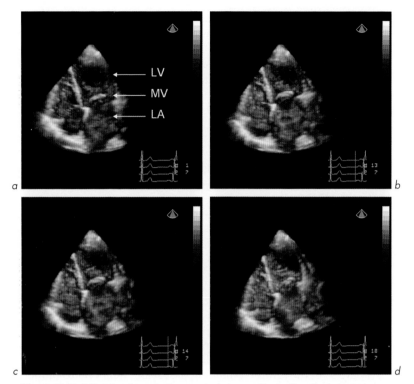

Figure 5.17 3-D echo. Images from a study in a patient with mitral stenosis.

reconstruction of congenital TV abnormalities such as AV canal defects and assessment of PV stenosis.
- Determination of the size of vegetations in endocarditis.

3. Congenital heart disease
- ASD. The size, shape and location of defects and their relationship to surrounding tissues and the extent of residual surrounding tissue can be assessed. In secundum ASDs, the extent of the retro-aortic rim often determines the feasibility of percutaneous device closure and 3-D echo can demonstrate successful closure.
- VSD. Visualization of the entire septum is an advantage to assess the size and shape of the defect and jet using colour flow techniques.
- LV and RV size and function can be assessed in patients with congenital heart disease.
- Circumferential extent of subaortic membranes can be visualized.
- Congenital valvular malformations (e.g. MV) can be examined.

4. Intraoperative

• MV prolapse repair, to assess anatomy, guide surgical repair and final adequacy of repair.
• Surgery for congenital heart lesions.
• HOCM during septal myomectomy to show the extent of septal thickening, LVOTO, MV SAM and post-procedure result.
• Guide catheters into the 3-D space without X-ray exposure, e.g. during EPS.

5. Aortic disease

• Define the anatomy of aortic dissection.

6. Contrast echo

• Improve quantification of LV volume and function.
• Evaluation of myocardial perfusion. Ability to record the entire LV and quantify the full extent of hypoperfused myocardium. The problem of microbubble destruction, even with triggered imaging, remains a challenge.

7. Tagging and tracking the LV surface in real-time

This helps in the quantification of myocardial mechanics and shows changes in regional shape and strain. The approach has potential and may have comparable uses and similar quantitative ability to cardiac MRI. The superior temporal resolution of echo should offer unique advantages. In the future, combining the greater temporal resolution of 3-D echo with the excellent spatial resolution of MRI or CT may yield excellent imaging techniques ('fusion imaging') providing anatomical and physiological information.

8. Teaching of cardiac anatomy and physiology, and research

Limitations of 3-D echo

There is great potential for 3-D echo, and techniques are becoming more widely used in clinical practice. However, there are some limitations:

• 3-D echo may only visualize what can also be seen on a good 2-D echo study. Thus, an expert echocardiographer may obtain similar information from a conventional examination without the need for costly instrumentation and long post-processing times
• Operator instruction and experience in 3-D echo is necessary
• 3-D echo image quality depends on the quality of 2-D images for the ability to obtain motion and artefact-free 3-D data
• 3-D echo can only create a virtual sense of depth on a flat 2-D screen

- Some 3-D echo techniques such as manual endocardial contour tracing and offline analysis are time-consuming
- Some of the technology remains expensive
- Size and weight of transducers can be high, although these are becoming more miniaturized.

Some of these limitations will be overcome with newer techniques. With rapid advances in digital image processing, 3-D echo is still in evolution. The incorporation of 3-D technology into conventional echo systems with operator-friendly applications is reducing the time and effort required to obtain 3-D images. Standard 3-D echo protocols are being developed. Further advances in real-time 3-D echo with real-time colour echo, contrast echo, tissue Doppler imaging and intracardiac ultrasound may be beneficial.

Ongoing and future developments in 3-D echo

These developments should increase the use of 3-D echo and make its use more routine. They include:

1. Technological advances (e.g. increased crystal density in transducers, improving resolution) and expanding clinical applications
2. Standardized 3-D study protocols, nomenclature and image displays
3. Automated surface detection and quantification
4. Single heartbeat full volume acquisition
5. Improvements in transthoracic and TOE real-time 3-D imaging
6. Transthoracic transducers are becoming smaller, almost to the size of 2-D, allowing 2-D and 3-D functions to be combined in one.

These and other echo techniques will undoubtedly find clinical use, but the existing echo techniques described in this book are very powerful and will continue to have important clinical uses.

5.5 ECHO IN SPECIAL HOSPITAL SETTINGS

Echo can be of great benefit in several special hospital situations:
- Preoperative
- Intraoperative
- Intensive care unit (ICU), coronary care unit (CCU), cardiac catheter laboratory
- Accident & Emergency (A&E) department
- Emergency echo
- Portable (hand-held) echo
- Intracardiac and intravascular ultrasound (IVUS).

PREOPERATIVE ECHO

Echo can help in the preoperative assessment of patients undergoing cardiac and non-cardiac surgery. There are internationally published guidelines including those by the American College of Cardiology, American Heart Association and European Society of Cardiology relating to echo assessment for preoperative patients. For non-cardiac surgery, particularly in high-risk operations such as orthopaedic or vascular surgery, echo can be used to assess LV systolic function or valvular function (see Box 5.2). Myocardial perfusion can be assessed by stress echo. Preoperative echo should be used for cardiac surgery (see Box 5.3) and for orthopaedic, vascular, major and genitourinary surgery.

Box 5.2 Cardiac risk for non-cardiac surgical procedures (death, MI)

High risk >5%

- Emergency major surgery, particularly in older people
- Aortic and other major vascular surgery
- Peripheral vascular surgery
- Anticipated prolonged surgery with significant blood loss and/or fluid shifts

Medium risk <5%

- Carotid endarterectomy
- Head and neck surgery
- Intraperitoneal surgery
- Intrathoracic surgery
- Orthopaedic surgery
- Urological surgery

Low risk <1%

- Endoscopic procedures
- Superficial procedures
- Cataract surgery
- Breast surgery

Adapted from Eagle KA, Berger PB, Calkins H, et al. ACC/AHA guideline update for perioperative cardiovascular evaluation for noncardiac surgery – executive summary. A report of the American College of Cardiology/American Heart Association Task Force on Practice Guidelines (Committee to Update the 1996 Guidelines on Perioperative Cardiovascular Evaluation for Noncardiac Surgery). Circulation. 2002;105:1257–1267.

Box 5.3 Clinical predictors of increased perioperative cardiovascular risk (death, MI, heart failure)

High risk

- Unstable coronary syndromes – recent (<30 days) or acute (<7 days) MI, unstable or severe angina (Canadian class III or IV)
- Decompensated heart failure
- Significant arrhythmia – high-level AV block, symptomatic ventricular arrhythmia with underlying heart disease, SVTs with poorly controlled ventricular rate
- Severe valvular abnormality

Medium risk

- Mild angina (Canadian class I or II)
- Previous MI
- Compensated or previous heart failure
- Diabetes mellitus
- Renal insufficiency

Low risk

- Advanced age
- Abnormal ECG – LVH, LBBB, ST-T abnormalities
- Low functional capacity
- Previous stroke
- Uncontrolled hypertension

Adapted from Eagle KA, Berger PB, Calkins H, et al. ACC/AHA guideline update for perioperative cardiovascular evaluation for noncardiac surgery – executive summary. A report of the American College of Cardiology/American Heart Association Task Force on Practice Guidelines (Committee to Update the 1996 Guidelines on Perioperative Cardiovascular Evaluation for Noncardiac Surgery). Circulation. 2002;105:1257–1267.

Specific uses of preoperative echo in cardiac and non-cardiac high-risk surgery

- Assessment of LV function – global, regional wall motion abnormalities, stress echo for demonstration of myocardial ischaemia
- MV assessment – need for valve operation and severity of MR or MS, suitability for MV repair, suitability for balloon valvuloplasty, mitral annular calcification
- AV assessment – AS and severity, suitability of AV replacement and prediction of annular size and LVOT size
- Pulmonary hypertension and right heart assessment
- Aortic atheroma
- Thoracic aortic aneurysm.

INTRAOPERATIVE ECHO

The use of intraoperative echo has increased in adult and paediatric surgery. This refers mainly to intraoperative TOE particularly for cardiac surgery, but this is also used in some high-risk non-cardiac operations. This technique can help in the acquisition of new information (12–38% of cases) during operation and may impact upon treatment (9–14% of cases).

Intraoperative TOE is not without risk and is an independent predictor of postoperative dysphagia (over 7 times greater odds in a study of 838 patients, but another study of 7200 patients showed no increased mortality and only 0.2% morbidity).

Uses of intraoperative TOE (from Cheitlin et al. 2003, ACC/AHA Practice Guidelines)

- MV repair. Detailed anatomical evaluation and adequacy of repair (residual MR, SAM and dynamic LVOTO, iatrogenic MS)
- MV replacement – valve sizing, adequacy or replacement, paravalvular MR (jets are more common after MV than AV replacements), chordal interference with valvular function
- Ventricular function – LV (regional, global) and RV
- AV replacement – valve sizing, adequacy of replacement, prosthesis size mismatch, paravalvular AR, LVOTO
- Congenital heart lesion repairs (e.g. transposition of the great arteries) – detection of residual defects after surgery, such as residual shunt, in 4.4–12.8% of cases, baffle interrogation, RV function
- Intracardiac air – intracavity, myocardial, adequacy of de-airing after bypass
- Surgical myomectomy for HOCM – residual LVOTO, acquired VSD, coronary fistula
- Aortic atheroma
- Minimally invasive cardiac surgery
- Coronary artery bypass surgery.

CORONARY CARE UNIT/INTENSIVE CARE UNIT/A&E/ CARDIAC CATHETER LABORATORY

There is a role for transthoracic echo and TOE. Examples include:
- Size of pericardial effusion, echo features of tamponade
- Pericardiocentesis – echo-guided assistance with placement of drainage catheter
- LV regional wall motion abnormalities in acute MI
- Valvular abnormalities

- Assessment of endocarditis or pyrexia of unknown origin (e.g. TOE to exclude endocarditis in an ICU patient with unexplained fever and *Staphylococcus aureus* in blood cultures)
- Assessment of the patient following major trauma
- Mitral balloon valvuloplasty
- Catheter placement during EPS and arrhythmia ablation.

EMERGENCY ECHO

The importance of echo in the management of critically ill patients is recognized (see Box 5.4). There may also be emergency situations when a full echo examination is not possible or necessary. A targeted (or focused) echo study may provide useful and potentially life-saving information to assist in the clinical assessment of a severely ill patient, where the clinical history and examination are paramount. Some training courses have been developed. For example, in the UK, the British Society of Echocardiography (BSE) and Resuscitation Council (UK) have produced the Focused Echocardiography in Emergency Life Support (FEEL) course (see Box 5.5). This is intended to train novice practitioners in TEE in the peri-resuscitation period and has been offered regularly since 2013. Each year, on average, 15 courses are held, training 200 healthcare professionals. The trainees are required to continue training locally by performing focused studies on critically ill patients under the supervision of a local mentor, before receiving accreditation. The scope of one such course is detailed in Box 5.5. Additionally, Critical Care Echocardiography Accreditation has been offered. In the UK, this is as a collaboration since 2012 between the BSE and the Intensive Care Society. Accreditation is also available under the direction of other national and international societies.

Box 5.4 Echo in emergency situations – underlying diagnoses and possible echo findings

Cardiac arrest – pulseless electrical activity (PEA)

- Cardiac tamponade – pericardial effusion, cardiac rupture, echo features of tamponade (e.g. RV and RA diastolic collapse)
- Massive pulmonary embolism (PE) – RV and RA dilatation, elevated PA systolic pressure
- Tension pneumothorax – heart may be obscured
- Anaphylactic shock/severe hypovolaemia – hyperdynamic LV, IVC collapse

---

Continued

Box 5.4 Echo in emergency situations – underlying diagnoses and possible echo findings—cont'd

Peri-cardiac arrest – resuscitated VF/VT

- Coronary artery disease (CAD) – reduced LVEF, regional wall motion abnormalities
- Valvular heart disease – severe AS, MS
- HCM/HOCM – LVOTO, SAM, ASH, LVH
- DCM (idiopathic or secondary – see Section 4.1) – dilated LV, reduced LVEF
- Arrhythmogenic cardiomyopathy – RV dilatation, RV dysplasia
- Idiopathic – echo may be normal (not during VF/VT)

Acute severe breathlessness

- LV systolic failure – reduced LVEF, severe valvular heart disease (e.g. AS, MS)
- PE – RV and RA dilatation, elevated PA systolic pressure
- Cardiac tamponade – pericardial effusion, cardiac rupture, echo features of tamponade (e.g. RV and RA diastolic collapse)
- Pneumonia – pleural and/or pericardial effusion
- Pleural effusion – effusion seen on echo (see Fig. 4.27)

Acute severe chest pain

- CAD – regional wall motion abnormalities, reduced LVEF
- PE – RV and RA dilatation, elevated PA systolic pressure
- Pericarditis – echo normal or pericardial effusion
- Aortic dissection* – dissection flap, aortic aneurysm, AR, pericardial effusion
- LVOTO – severe AS, HOCM
- Pneumonia – pleural and/or pericardial effusion

Severe hypotension

- Cardiogenic shock – reduced LVEF, reduced RVEF, severe AS, severe MS, acute severe MR or AR, cardiac tamponade, post-MI VSD
- PE – RV and RA dilatation, elevated PA systolic pressure
- Anaphylactic shock/severe hypovolaemia – hyperdynamic LV, IVC collapse
- Cardiac tamponade – pericardial effusion, cardiac rupture, echo features of tamponade (e.g. RV and RA diastolic collapse)

Continued

Box 5.4 Echo in emergency situations – underlying diagnoses and possible echo findings—cont'd

Blunt trauma

- Myocardial contusion – reduced LVEF, regional wall motion abnormalities, pericardial effusion
- Coronary artery injury/damage – reduced LVEF, regional wall motion abnormality, pericardial effusion
- Cardiac rupture – pericardial effusion, cardiac tamponade
- Aortic dissection or rupture* – dissection flap, aortic aneurysm, AR, pericardial effusion
- Valvular abnormality/dysfunction – leaflet tear, AR, MR, TR, PR, chordal or papillary muscle rupture.

*Best seen using TOE.

Box 5.5 FEEL (UK) course is run by the British Society of Echocardiography (BSE) and the Resuscitation Council (UK)

Intended for healthcare professionals involved in the care of critically ill patients.

Does not require any previous echo or ultrasound experience.

Intended as an adjunct to advanced life support (ALS), and knowledge of the current ALS algorithm is required.

FEEL course teaches the knowledge and skills required to:
- Achieve 4 standard TTE views: parasternal long-axis (PLAX), parasternal short-axis (PSAX), apical 4-chamber (A4C) and subcostal (SC)
- Perform ALS-conformed echo: synchronized with pulse checks thus limiting no-flow intervals during CPR
- Interpret images and diagnose potentially treatable causes of cardiac arrest/circulatory collapse:
  - Severe myocardial insufficiency (including acute MI)
  - Pericardial collection (PC) – massive
  - Pulmonary embolism (PE) – massive
  - Severe hypovolaemia
  - Tension pneumothorax
  - Exclude VF
- Communicate with the resuscitation team
- Understand the pitfalls and limitations of focused echo
- Understand the requirements and mechanisms for ongoing training and certification in peri-resuscitation echo
- Understand the importance of clinical governance with respect to emergency echo

Adapted from information from the Resuscitation Council (UK) website at <http://www.resus.org.uk/information-on-courses/focused-echocardiography-in-emergency-life-support/>.

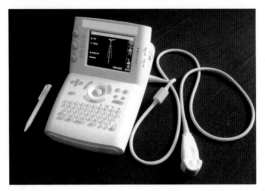

Figure 5.18 Portable echocardiogram machine. The mass is under 3 kg. Pen shown for scale is 14 cm long.

PORTABLE OR HAND-HELD ECHO

This refers to the use of small, lightweight, portable echo machines, which can be used in different locations at the patient's bedside (Fig. 5.18). These vary in their levels of complexity from very simple pocket-size instruments to larger instruments the size of a laptop computer or briefcase with many features of larger machines. Some have limited capability with a single transducer producing 2-D images and others have more modalities including 2-D, M-mode, pulsed wave and continuous wave Doppler and colour flow imaging. Some support multiple echo transducers and have sophisticated functions such as TOE. These instruments can be used in situations such as the A&E department, CCU and cardiology outpatients clinic. Some devices will operate from a battery source and can be used outside the hospital, for example, at the scene of a trauma incident. There needs to be careful local evaluation of the clinical indications and quality assurance in the use of these devices in each medical centre, to monitor diagnostic accuracy.

Clinical uses of portable echo

- Rapid assessment of patients in the A&E department, ICU, CCU and cardiac catheter laboratory
- Exclusion of pericardial effusion and/or echo features of tamponade in trauma patients
- Assessment of LV and RV systolic function
- Regional wall motion abnormalities
- Identification of valvular abnormalities such as AS or MR
- Assessment of patients with hypertension to determine if there is LVH
- Assessment of patients with chest pain and non-diagnostic ECG where an akinetic LV segment may indicate acute MI, whereas a pericardial effusion may indicate pericarditis

- Assessment of patients with hypotension, where a small hyperdynamic LV may suggest septicaemic shock whilst a dilated poor LV may suggest a primary cardiac abnormality
- Portable echo can in some situations be a useful supplement to the physical examination.

Limitations of portable echo

- Appropriate training and experience are needed for any echo assessment
- Misdiagnosis due to the limitation of instruments giving suboptimal image quality and inexperienced operator
- If an abnormality is suggested then a full echo examination may be needed with standard equipment.

INTRACARDIAC ECHO

This uses a catheter-like ultrasound probe which is passed to the right heart from the femoral vein. The frequency used is 5–10 MHz. This allows ultrasound penetration of tissues up to 10 cm from the transducer. At present, devices provide single-plane imaging with pulsed wave and colour Doppler using a steerable transducer connected to standard echo equipment.

The tip of the transducer can be placed in the IVC, RA and RV. The RA is often the most useful location for monitoring invasive procedures. From the RA, it is possible to obtain echo views of the AV, MV, TV, LV and RV, as well as the interatrial septum, LA and pulmonary veins. From the IVC the transducer can be used to visualize the abdominal aorta.

Clinical uses of intracardiac echo

This is used primarily for monitoring invasive procedures in the cardiac catheter laboratory, although the clinical utility of this technique has not been fully evaluated. Intracardiac echo may be used because the image quality with transthoracic is usually suboptimal in these situations. It may be used as an alternative to TOE during invasive procedures, as TOE often requires general anaesthesia because of the duration of the procedure. Intracardiac echo is well tolerated and provides accurate continuous information to the physician carrying out the procedure.

The primary applications of intracardiac echo are in monitoring during:

- Percutaneous device closure of defects (e.g. ASD)
- Balloon valvuloplasty (e.g. MS)
- Electrophysiological studies (EPS) (e.g. catheter ablation procedures for arrhythmias).

For device closures, this technique can be used to evaluate the defect at baseline and identify adjacent structures such as pulmonary veins. During the procedure, the technique can be used to help position the closure device optimally. After the procedure, Doppler and colour flow mapping can be used to examine for any residual shunt.

In EPS, intracardiac echo can be used to:

- Monitor trans-septal puncture
- Give detailed evaluation of LA and pulmonary vein anatomy
- Allow placement of the ablation probe with optimum tissue contact
- Monitor the development of spontaneous echo contrast during ablation
- Detect complications such as intracardiac thrombus, pericardial effusion or pulmonary vein obstruction.

Limitations of intracardiac echo

- Cost. Disposable catheters are expensive
- Risks of invasive procedure. However, most patients are already having an invasive procedure and there is a little additional risk
- Image quality. Bi-plane or multi-plane probes will improve image acquisition.

INTRAVASCULAR ULTRASOUND (IVUS)

This is performed using an intravascular steerable catheter that is positioned within the coronary arteries during interventional coronary procedures. The ultrasound frequency used is 30–50 MHz. The transducer provides an image depth of 2–3 cm with high resolution into the vessel wall and atherosclerotic plaques. A small dedicated ultrasound system is usually used to acquire the images. The catheter is positioned by the interventional cardiologist during the procedure.

IVUS may be useful when standard angiographic data do not give full information regarding the length or severity of a coronary artery narrowing and the condition of the atherosclerotic plaque. This information can then be used to plan further treatment.

CARDIAC MASSES, INFECTION, CONGENITAL ABNORMALITIES AND AORTA

6.1 CARDIAC MASSES

Echo is very important in detecting cardiac masses and giving an indication of their nature. Masses include:

- Tumours (primary or secondary)
- Blood clot (thrombus)
- Infected material (vegetation or abscess)
- Artificial (prosthetic) valves and pacing wires.

1. TUMOURS OF THE HEART

Echo can detect the site, size, mobility, number and attachment of tumours. This is especially helpful when planning surgical treatment.

Secondary tumours – the majority

These are all malignant since they have metastasized or invaded locally. They are more common than generally realized, occurring in about 10% of all fatal malignancies. The most common primary site is the lung (30% of cases of cardiac secondaries – the close proximity plays a role with direct extension to involve the pericardium and heart). Other common primary tumours metastasizing to the heart include breast, kidney, liver, melanoma (this is disproportionately numerous in relation to its total incidence), lymphoma and leukaemia.

Primary tumours – rare

Benign. For example, myxoma, lipoma, fibroma, rhabdomyoma, papillary fibroelastoma, angioma, paraganglioma and pericardial tumours (pericardial cysts and teratomas).

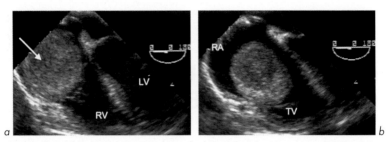

Figure 6.1 (a) Leiomyosarcoma (arrow) of the inferior vena cava extending into the right atrium. **(b)** The mass prolapses through the tricuspid valve. TOE 4-chamber view.

Malignant. Mainly sarcomas, e.g. angiosarcoma (most common), rhabdomyosarcoma, fibrosarcoma and liposarcoma.

Echo cannot differentiate between benign and malignant tumours. **2-D echo** shows tumours as echogenic masses within the cavity of the heart, attached to the wall or in the pericardium. The size and mobility can be determined. As with all echo studies, multiple views should be obtained. Occasionally on **M-mode**, a tumour such as myxoma may be seen interfering with valve function (Section 2.1). The effects of tumours (e.g. obstruction of valve flow, LV dysfunction due to infiltration or obstruction or pericardial effusion) can also be seen on echo (Fig. 6.1).

Myxoma

Myxomas are rare and occur in the atria or ventricles. They are gelatinous and friable (bits can break away and embolize).
• Single or rarely multiple
• Any age or sex but most common in middle-aged women
• Most commonly in LA (3 times more common than RA) attached to foramen ovale margin (>80%) and rarely in RV or LV
• The myxoma has a base that is either thin like a stalk or broad
• Myxomas are always attached to either the interatrial or interventricular septum.

Although benign in the neoplastic sense, they are far from benign in their effects. They are slow growing over years and, if untreated, are usually fatal.

The effects of myxomas relate to:
• Local cardiac effects (e.g. obstruction of MV, which can be sudden and fatal)
• Thromboembolic effects
• Neoplastic effects – fever (pyrexia of unknown origin), weight loss, anaemia, arthralgia, Raynaud's phenomenon, high erythrocyte sedimentation rate (ESR).

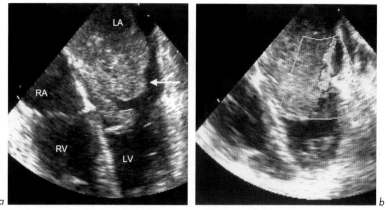

a   b

Figure 6.2 (a) Left atrial myxoma (arrow) shown on TOE 4-chamber view. The tumour is large and lobulated with a broad base attaching it to the interatrial septum. It can be seen to prolapse through the mitral valve. **(b)** It is producing a marked space-occupying effect and causing restriction of flow within the left atrium.

Myxomas usually present in one of four ways, in decreasing order of frequency:

1. Breathlessness
2. Systemic emboli
3. Constitutional upset
4. Sudden death (occlusion of MV orifice).

Myxomas may be readily detected by **M-mode** or **2-D echo** (Fig. 6.2). The myxoma can be seen as a mass in the LA cavity and may prolapse through the MV into the LV cavity during diastole obstructing flow. It may be so large as to fill the LA. **Doppler** can show the haemodynamic effects.

Myxomas very rarely occur in an autosomal-dominant familial fashion associated with lentiginosis (multiple freckles) or HCM and so it is wise to screen all first-degree relatives by echo (Section 7.6).

Pericardial cysts

These are the most common primary pericardial tumours and are often detected in middle age as an incidental finding during chest X-ray or echo performed for another indication. They can occur anywhere in the pericardium and are masses with echo-free centres attached to the pericardium and with intact walls separating them from the LV cavity. They are benign.

Pericardial fat pad

Adipose tissue (fat) may be present between the pericardium and epicardium. This has a granular, speckled appearance on echo. It is more commonly found in older people and people with obesity or diabetes.

2. THROMBUS

This may occur in the ventricular or atrial cavities or walls (mural thrombus). Situations where thrombus formation is increased:
• Dilatation of cardiac chambers
• Reduced wall contractility
• Obstruction and stagnation of flow.

Some examples of these situations include:
• Dilated cardiomyopathy
• Following MI
• LV aneurysm
• LA in valve disease (e.g. MS)
• Prosthetic valves
• Arrhythmia (e.g. AF).

2-D imaging is the best echo technique to identify thrombus, which is usually echo-bright. However, this is not always the case and it can be difficult to distinguish from myocardium if they have similar echogenicity. TOE can be helpful, especially for LA and LA appendage thrombus.
    False-positive identification of thrombus may occur due to:
• Localized increase in wall thickness
• Tumours
• Dense echoes due to stagnation of blood in an enlarged chamber.

The following favour the diagnosis of thrombus:
1. Mural thrombus may be distinguished from myocardium since myocardium thickens during systole and thrombus does not.
2. Wall motion near a thrombus is nearly always abnormal whereas it is often normal near other pathology (e.g. a tumour).
3. Thrombus usually has a clear identifiable edge, which distinguishes it from wall artefact or hazy stagnant blood.
4. Colour flow mapping can distinguish thrombus from stagnant flow.

Several echo views should always be taken. On 2-D echo, thrombus may be seen as a ball-like or a frond-like mass, or as a well-organized, laminated, raised thickening in the LA or LV. In the LA, there may be associated evidence of sluggish blood flow such as 'spontaneous contrast'. The LA appendage may contain thrombus which can be identified on TOE (Figs. 5.7, 6.3).

6.2 INFECTION

ENDOCARDITIS

This refers to inflammation of any part of the inner layer of the heart, the endocardium, including the heart valves. Inflammatory and/or

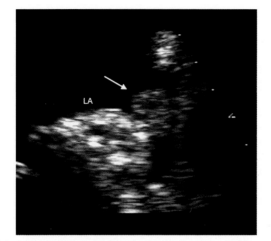

Figure 6.3 Left atrial appendage thrombus (arrow) seen on TOE.

infected material may accumulate on valves to cause masses called 'vegetations'. These are made up of a mixture of infective material, thrombus, fibrin and red and white blood cells. Vegetations are usually attached on valves but may be on other locations, e.g. chordae, LA, LVOT (HCM), right side of VSD (jet lesion).

The size of vegetations varies from <1 mm to several centimetres. TTE can miss vegetations of <2 mm. TOE may show these, and improves sensitivity to >85%. Large vegetations are particularly associated with fungal infection or endocarditis of the TV. Vegetations may be detected by M-mode (Section 2.1) or 2-D techniques where they are seen as mobile echo-reflective masses.

There are several potential causes that may be infective or non-infective.

Infective
- Bacterial – *Streptococcus*, *Staphylococcus*, Gram-negative bacteria, etc.
- Fungal – *Aspergillus*, *Candida*
- Other – *Chlamydia*, *Coxiella*.

Non-infective
- Associated with malignancy (marantic)
- Connective tissue disease – SLE (Libman–Sacks), rheumatoid arthritis
- Acute rheumatic fever (with associated myocarditis and pericarditis).

It is not possible to distinguish by echo alone between infective and non-infective vegetations.

Infective endocarditis

Infection may occur on normal native valves, on previously diseased valves (e.g. rheumatic valves or calcified, degenerative valves) or on artificial (prosthetic) valves.

Endocarditis is a serious condition and potentially life-threatening. It can be acute (e.g. with *Staphylococcus aureus*) or subacute bacterial (SBE). Infection usually follows an episode of bacteraemia, which may not be readily identifiable, or may follow dental treatment or surgery. For this reason, it is safest to advise antibiotic prophylaxis treatment for all dental treatment and all surgical procedures for people with a known cardiac murmur (refer to local guidelines, which vary internationally), congenital lesion, heart valve abnormality or artificial valve. Certain infecting organisms are associated with underlying disease conditions (e.g. *Streptococcus bovis* endocarditis with carcinoma of the colon).

Remember that endocarditis is a *clinical* diagnosis made on the basis of clinical history and examination, blood tests suggesting inflammation and immune complex phenomena and, if possible, culture of the organism from blood. The absence of vegetations on an echo does *not* exclude the diagnosis of endocarditis suspected on clinical grounds. Endocarditis may be present even in the absence of a murmur or fever, especially if antibiotics have been given.

Clinical features supporting endocarditis

- Infection – fever, malaise, night sweats, rigors, anaemia, splenomegaly, clubbing
- Immune complex deposition – microscopic haematuria, vasculitic skin and retinal lesions
- Emboli – in distant organs (brain, retinal, coronary, splenic, renal, femoropopliteal, mesenteric), which may lead to abscess formation
- Cardiac complications:
  1. New or changing murmur(s)
  2. Valve destruction causing regurgitation
  3. Abscess formation around valve rings or in septum causing heart block
  4. Aortic root abscesses that may produce sinus of Valsalva aneurysm or involve coronary ostia
  5. Large vegetations that may obstruct valves (e.g. aortic fungal endocarditis)
  6. Heart failure that may be fatal – due to involvement of the myocardium, pericardial effusion, pyopericardium (pus in the pericardial space, a very serious situation) or valve dysfunction.

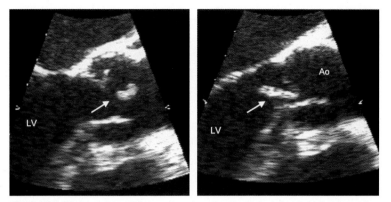

Figure 6.4 Endocarditis of the aortic valve showing a large vegetation (arrow). TOE images.

Important investigations in endocarditis

• Blood cultures – at least 3 sets from 3 different sites at different times. Up to 90% will be culture positive
• Blood count – raised neutrophil count, normochromic normocytic anaemia
• ESR and C-reactive protein – raised markers of inflammation. Fall accompanies response to treatment
• Immune complex titres raised
• Low complement concentrations
• Urine microscopy – microscopic haematuria
• ECG – lengthening of the PR interval suggests aortic root and septal abscess
• Echo – TTE and/or TOE (Figs. 6.4, 6.8).

Cardiac lesions predisposing to endocarditis

1. Common

• Native valve disease – AV (bicuspid, rheumatic, calcific), MV (regurgitation more often than stenosis, MV prolapse)
• Prosthetic valves
• TV in intravenous drug abusers or after intravenous cannulation (especially large veins)
• Congenital – aortic coarctation, PDA, VSD.

2. Uncommon

• Previously normal valves
• HCM and subaortic stenosis
• Mural thrombus

- Jet lesion
- AV fistula.

3. Rare (virtually never)

- ASD
- Pulmonary stenosis
- Divided PDA.

Antibiotic prophylaxis to prevent endocarditis

The recommended use of prophylaxis and the antibiotic regimen should be checked locally – as there are regional variations – and must include attention to a patient's known antibiotic allergies. May be used in:

- Prosthetic valve
- Previous endocarditis
- Prevention of recurrence of rheumatic fever
- Known cardiac valve lesion
- Congenital cardiac abnormality – septal defect, PDA.

For:
1. Dental treatment
2. Genitourinary procedures
3. Upper respiratory tract procedures
4. Obstetric, gynaecological and gastrointestinal procedures.

Uses of echo in endocarditis

- Aid diagnosis
- Detect predisposing lesions
- Search for complications
- Response to treatment
- Timing surgical intervention if necessary.

Remember that many vegetations are not seen on TTE until they are >2 mm in size. Colour Doppler may identify AR or MR, acquired VSD or a septal abscess. TOE is very useful in endocarditis, particularly for:

- Visualizing small vegetations
- MV
- Prosthetic valve endocarditis
- Leaflet perforation
- Aortic root abscess
- Sinus of Valsalva aneurysm
- LVOT aneurysm
- LVOT to RA fistula.

Evaluating response to treatment – role for serial echo?

How often serial echos should be done is not clear-cut. Some centres perform weekly echos whilst antibiotics are being given. It is difficult to justify this routinely unless it will alter clinical management. Echo can be carried out if there is a deterioration in clinical state of the patient. Vegetations that become smaller may indicate response to treatment – or this may indicate reduced mobility or embolization of part or all of the vegetation! Vegetations getting bigger or new complications (e.g. abscess formation) indicate persistent infection or ineffective treatment.

Timing surgery

Treatment of endocarditis is with antibiotics, usually given for an empirically determined time period of 6 weeks. If an organism is identified, antibiotic therapy can be tailored with known sensitivities. Surgery may be necessary for complications, such as valvular regurgitation or abscess formation. Embolization of infected material may cause cerebral abscesses, which need special treatment (antibiotics and surgical drainage).

Echo may detect some indications for surgery in endocarditis

This is not a clear-cut decision and should be based on clinical grounds:
- AR or MR not responding to treatment
- Sinus of Valsalva aneurysm
- Aortic root and septal abscess
- Valve obstruction due to large vegetations
- Failure of antibiotics to control infection or relapse of infection despite changes in antibiotics
- Fungal endocarditis (usually responds best to valve replacement and antifungal treatment)
- Large vegetations with embolic phenomena
- Prosthetic valve endocarditis (usually required).

Consequences and complications of infection

- Spread of vegetations onto other valves or structures (e.g. chordae)
- Valvular regurgitation – rupture, prolapse or perforation of valve leaflets or abscess causing regurgitation
- Abscess formation – echo-free space in the perivalvular area (especially AV), which may cause sinus of Valsalva rupture and left-to-right shunting (often aortic to RA). Abscess in the IVS may cause heart block (usually aortic endocarditis).

Prosthetic valve endocarditis

This can occur on tissue or mechanical valves. Echo can be difficult because of the artefact (reverberation and masking) caused by the prosthesis. It may show vegetations, the complications of infection (e.g. regurgitation) or abscess. TOE may be helpful in making the diagnosis. Endocarditis affecting prosthetic valves is very serious and further valve surgery is often required (see Section 6.3).

6.3 ARTIFICIAL (PROSTHETIC) VALVES

These have been used to replace diseased native valves since the 1960s. Although such surgery is still common, attempts are now often made by surgeons to repair valves (particularly the MV) rather than replace them, where possible.

Valves can be positioned to replace any of the 4 native valves. Some patients have more than one prosthetic valve. They may be made of:
- Biological tissue from human or animal valves
- Non-valve tissue material (e.g. pericardium)
- Inert non-biological materials (plastic, metal, carbon, fabric).

A combination of biological tissue and inert material is sometimes used (Fig. 6.5).
1. **Mechanical valves** – anticoagulation with an agent such as warfarin is necessary to prevent thrombosis:
   - Ball and cage (e.g. Starr–Edwards)
   - Tilting disc – one cusp (e.g. Björk–Shiley) or two cusps (e.g. St Jude).
2. **Tissue (biological) valves**
   - Heterograft – from animals
     Porcine – from pigs. Less thrombogenic but less durable than mechanical valves (stenosis or regurgitation usually in 10–15 years). Often have 3 cusps, made of biological tissue fixed by 3 metal stents to a metal sewing ring (e.g. Carpentier–Edwards).
     Bovine – from cattle. Not commonly used (e.g. Ionescu–Shiley valve [bovine pericardial leaflets and titanium frame])
   - Homograft – from humans
     Initially, their lifetime was limited (3 years) but better preservation techniques (e.g. cryopreservation) have increased their usefulness.

ECHO EXAMINATION OF PROSTHETIC VALVES

Echo can assess:
1. Anatomy – calcification, degeneration, seated correctly or rocking
2. Function:
   - Obstruction – all have some degree of stenosis but this can increase in malfunctioning valves

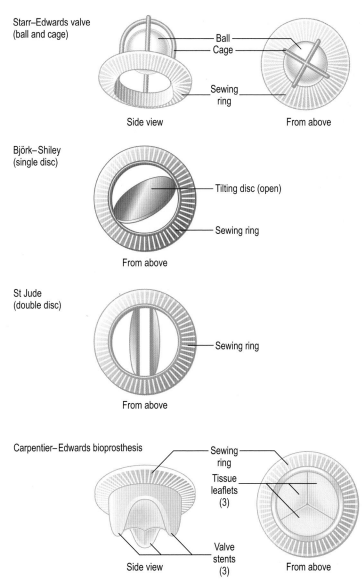

Figure 6.5 Prosthetic heart valves.

• Regurgitation – through valve orifice or paravalvular (due to infection or rocking due to loosening of stitching or degeneration)
3. Infection – valvular, paravalvular abscess
4. Thrombosis.

Examination can be difficult because prosthetic valves:
• Have varied and specialized structures
• Are usually highly echogenic (especially mechanical valves). They may produce echo artefacts such as very bright echo reflection (termed reverberation). They also cast an acoustic shadow that masks or obscures deeper structures.

Following valve replacement surgery, a baseline echo study is often performed after a few weeks. Serial examinations may be performed at intervals after surgery (Section 7.6). The type and size of valve should be on the echo request form. As indicated earlier, TOE is an important supplement to TTE in examining prosthetic valves.

M-mode can give some characteristic appearances:
• A Starr–Edwards valve typically shows 2 dense, almost parallel, echo lines representing the sewing ring and the cage. Only echo reflections from the anterior surface of the ball are seen and are traced as dense lines. In the open position, the reflection from the ball moves as far as the cage line and never beyond. In the closed position, the echo line from the cage is recorded halfway between the cage and sewing ring in an almost parallel position.

Reverberations are seen below the valve tracings representing echo reflections from the posterior surface of the ball.
• A St Jude valve in the open position shows parallel lines of the disc parallel to the sewing ring. In the closed position, no echo lines are recorded (the disc lies within the sewing ring).
• In biological prostheses, the sewing ring is seen as a continuous echo line. Leaflets show echo tracings similar to native valves, with a leaflet excursion giving a box-like shape. Echo lines representing 2 of the 3 stents may be seen.

2-D echo gives important anatomical information. If no surgical operative details are available, some aspects of the echo examination may help to identify which type of valve is present (it is easier to make this assessment for mitral [Fig. 6.6] than aortic valves):
• Ball and cage – characteristic semi-circular echo image of the cage with the ball moving up and down
• Tilting disc – the movement of one or two discs can be seen opening and closing
• Tissue – the metal stents can often be seen in the LV cavity (mitral) or aorta (aortic).

Doppler echo is very useful in evaluating prosthetic valve function:

Obstruction to flow
Because of the non-compliant nature of the material in these valves, velocity of flow through them has a different range from normal

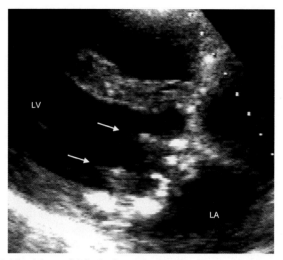

Figure 6.6 Mitral tissue (biological) prosthetic valve. Parasternal long-axis view showing the normal appearance of 2 of the supporting stents (arrows) within the left ventricular cavity.

Table 6.1 Velocity of flow (m/s) through some normally functioning mechanical and tissue prosthetic valves

Valve	Mitral	Aortic
Ball and cage Starr–Edwards	1.4–2.2	2.6–3.0
Single disc Björk–Shiley	1.3–1.8	1.9–2.9
Double disc St Jude	1.2–1.8	2.3–2.8
Porcine biological Carpentier–Edwards	1.5–2.0	1.9–2.8

native valves (see Table 6.1). Most prosthetic valves give some obstruction to flow. A number of measurements can be made:

1. *Peak velocity.* This is higher than in normal valves because of the relatively smaller orifice area caused by the bulk of the artificial material. An example of the range is given in Table 6.1.

   As a general rule of thumb, a peak velocity of >2 m/s in the MV usually indicates dysfunction in both mechanical and biological prosthetic valves. Aortic prosthesis flow velocity is normally <3 m/s.

2. *Pressure gradient* (ΔP). This is calculated by the simplified Bernoulli equation ($\Delta P = 4V^2$).

3. *Valve orifice area* – is measured using the continuity equation (see Chapter 3).

Different echo laboratories have different ranges. A change in velocity from postoperative values is more important in an individual case.

Regurgitation

This may be through the valve orifice (transvalvular) or around the sewing ring (paraprosthetic). Mild transvalvular MR can be found in normally functioning valves, more often in mechanical valves. This is due to valve closure or through the gaps between different parts of the prosthesis. It can be difficult to detect this due to masking. Moderate or severe MR is abnormal.

Continuous wave Doppler is more useful than pulsed wave and **colour flow** is good for showing anterograde and retrograde flows. Turbulent forward flow is shown as a mosaic of colours. In mitral bioprostheses one jet is usually seen. In most mitral mechanical valves, 2 jets are seen (almost equal size in Starr–Edwards, one smaller than the other in Björk–Shiley valves).

In regurgitation (Fig. 6.7), there may be a number of jets of different sizes depending on valve type (e.g. 2 jets in Björk–Shiley, multiple in Starr–Edwards). Colour flow also helps in differentiating between transvalvular and paravalvular regurgitation and helps to show new regurgitation.

PROSTHETIC VALVE MALFUNCTION

A false diagnosis of malfunction may be made if there is a low cardiac output, arrhythmia such as AV block or poor surgical technique

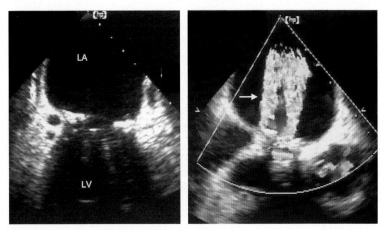

Figure 6.7 Regurgitation through a Starr–Edwards mitral valve prosthesis. Two jets can be seen on TOE with colour flow Doppler – a transvalvular jet and a paraprosthetic jet (arrow).

(e.g. valve that is too small or too large for the heart). Types of malfunction include:
- In mechanical and biological valves: endocarditis, dehiscence (valve becomes loose or detached), regurgitation
- More common in mechanical valves: thrombus, variance (change in shape or size)
- More common in biological valves: degeneration – stenosis or regurgitation.

ECHO FEATURES OF VALVE MALFUNCTION

Findings should be compared with baseline values where possible.
1. Anatomical abnormalities of prosthesis (by M-mode and 2-D echo):
   - Loose part of valve (e.g. ruptured bioprosthesis leaflet)
   - Loose sutures
   - Abnormal motion – reduced or exaggerated motion of any part of prosthesis
   - Associated findings, e.g. calcification, thrombus, vegetation, abscess, increased chamber size (LV, LA).
2. Haemodynamic abnormalities of prosthesis (by Doppler and colour flow):
   - Obstruction may be suggested by increased flow velocity or reduced orifice area
   - Regurgitation – increased severity of jet or new jet.

ENDOCARDITIS OF PROSTHETIC VALVES

This is a very serious problem and often results in a need for the valve to be surgically replaced, often after a period of treatment with intravenous antibiotics. Antibiotic prophylaxis for all dental treatment and surgery is essential to try to prevent this. Endocarditis can affect mechanical or biological prostheses. It occurs at an annual rate of 3–5% in people with prosthetic valves.

The following are suggestive findings:
- Vegetations (mobile masses on valve, move in cardiac cycle, but are often difficult to see)
- Incomplete valve closure due to interference by vegetations with valve leaflets
- Abscess seen as poorly echo-reflective areas around sewing ring
- Sutures may be seen moving freely if dehiscence occurs.

M-mode may show vegetations as multiple thick echo lines superimposed on M-mode of prosthesis, but both **M-mode** and **2-D echo** may be difficult because of reverberations and masking. Small vegetations (<2–3 mm) may be missed. It can be difficult sometimes to distinguish vegetations from calcified or thickened leaflets.

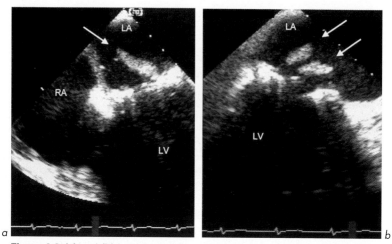

Figure 6.8 (a) and **(b)** Large vegetations (arrows) seen on TOE on the atrial side of a Starr–Edwards mitral valve prosthesis.

Doppler and **colour flow** can show haemodynamic consequences of endocarditis – transvalvular regurgitation (vegetations affecting leaflet closure), paravalvular regurgitation (abscess formation at suture lines), or increased forwards flow due to obstruction by vegetation. As mentioned, TOE is very useful in these situations (Fig. 6.8).

THROMBUS

More common in mechanical valves and responsible for many cases of malfunction. This can occur if anticoagulation control is poor or in the presence of dilated cardiac chambers.

Anticoagulation is essential for all mechanical valves (aim for international normalized ratio [INR] of 3.5–5.0). The susceptibility of prosthetic valves to thrombosis depends on their position (related to the pressure gradient across the valve):

tricuspid > mitral > pulmonary > aortic.

Sometimes, patients complain that they can no longer hear the valve clicking – this may be an indication of thrombosis.

Echo can detect thrombus by:

- Visualization of a mobile mass on the valve – it can be difficult to distinguish from vegetations or calcified nodules
- Reduced or absent motion of the mobile part of the valve (e.g. ball, disc, cusps)
- Associated dilatation of cardiac chambers.

As with vegetations, **M-mode** may show multiple dark echo lines and/or reduced valve opening or closing. **Doppler** and **colour flow** may show obstruction of valve opening (increased flow velocity) or obstruction of closure (a new transvalvular regurgitant jet or increase in severity of existing regurgitation).

DEHISCENCE

This is the failure of the sutures to attach the valve ring to the surrounding native tissues because of either loosening or rupture of one or more sutures. This may result in paravalvular regurgitation and/or abnormal valve motion (e.g. valve rocking or sutures may be seen moving freely).

REGURGITATION

Transvalvular. A mild degree is often seen as part of the normal function of the valve. It is increased by any factor that causes incomplete closure of prosthetic valves (e.g. vegetation, thrombus, variance or degeneration). It can be detected by colour flow or continuous wave Doppler.

Paravalvular. This is abnormal. It can be caused by endocarditis (abscess), dehiscence or other causes. Colour flow will show a regurgitant jet through an area outside the sewing ring.

VARIANCE

This is less common with the newer mechanical valves. It is a change in the shape and size of a mechanical valve due to erosions or cracks in the body of the ball or the disc or deposition of material into the valve (e.g. fibrous tissue or lipids onto the ball or metallic surface of the prosthesis).

The ball or disc becomes larger or smaller causing obstruction or incomplete closure, respectively. Echo can detect reduced motion of the ball or disc, increased flow velocity or transvalvular regurgitation.

DEGENERATION

Degeneration occurs in most biological prostheses within a few years. This leads to calcification and stenosis and/or rupture of valve leaflets and regurgitation towards the end of the expected lifespan of the valve. Echo may show calcification, abnormal leaflet motion and/or regurgitation.

6.4 CONGENITAL ABNORMALITIES

Echo is essential in the diagnosis of congenital heart disease and has reduced the need for cardiac catheterization in such conditions. Echo allows anatomical and haemodynamic assessment (e.g. the location and size of shunts, cardiac chamber anatomy and connections, and pressures such as pulmonary artery pressure).

1. SHUNTS

The term 'cardiac shunt' describes the flow of blood through an abnormal communication between different cardiac chambers or blood vessels. Examples of such communications are ASD, VSD or PDA. Blood will flow from a region of higher pressure to a region of lower pressure, usually left to right (e.g. LV to RV across a VSD). This results in increased blood flow and raised pressures on the right heart. Untreated, this can lead to right heart dilatation and failure. In some cases, irreversible changes in the pulmonary vasculature occur and the resistance in these vessels increases. This raises right-sided pressures with PHT (**Eisenmenger reaction** – the combination of a shunt with PHT), which may exceed left-sided pressures. 'Shunt reversal' then occurs (right-to-left shunting). This causes central cyanosis as deoxygenated blood enters the systemic circulation.

The larger the size of the shunt (the more blood passing across an abnormal communication), the more likely it is to be haemodynamically significant and require closure of the defect. Note that when the Eisenmenger reaction has occurred, it is usually too late to close a defect safely, since right heart failure may occur and is often fatal.

VSD, ASD, PFO (Figs. 6.9, 6.10, 6.11)

Defects may be identified in the ventricular or atrial septa by 2-D studies. The direction of flow across such defects can be shown by colour flow mapping and the velocity of the jet across the defect can be measured (and hence the pressure gradient identified) by continuous wave Doppler. This is especially useful in VSDs where a high-velocity jet suggests a high-pressure gradient between LV and RV and is referred to as a restrictive VSD. This is less likely to have a large shunt. VSD can occur in the upper membranous or lower muscular septum.

The interatrial septum (IAS) is often thin and in certain views in normal individuals (especially the apical 4-chamber view) there can appear to be a defect in a normal septum, giving the false illusion of an ASD. This is due to an effect known as 'echo drop-out', which happens because the reflected echo signal from the IAS is weak. The IAS in this view is being hit along its edge by the ultrasound beam and is at a large depth from the transducer. By examining the IAS from other views (e.g. subcostal), it can be seen that it is intact.

TOE allows excellent visualization of IAS and hence diagnosis of ASD (Figs. 5.12, 6.12, 6.13) and PFO. It can detect the size, number and type (location) of ASD, and suitability for percutaneous catheter-guided device closure rather than surgery.

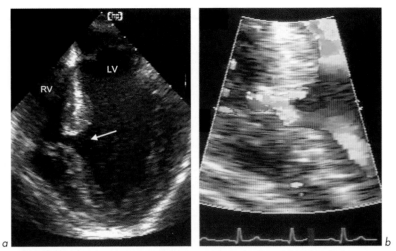

Figure 6.9 (a) Muscular ventricular septal defect (arrow). **(b)** Colour flow mapping shows flow from left to right ventricle.

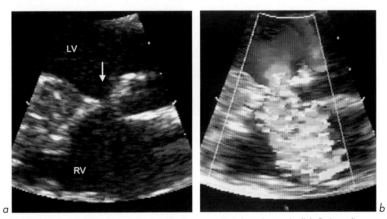

Figure 6.10 (a) Membranous ventricular septal defect (arrow). **(b)** Colour flow from left to right ventricle.

Currently, **device closure for ASD** is suitable if:
- Not multiple
- Not too close to MV or TV
- Size <30 mm.

TTE and TOE are both good at diagnosing ostium primum ASDs but TOE is better than TTE in diagnosing secundum ASDs under 10 mm in diameter. Defects of under 5 mm are only diagnosed correctly by TTE 20% of the time. 5–10 mm secundum ASDs are detected by TTE in 80% of cases.

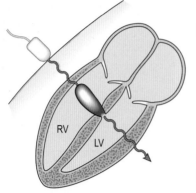

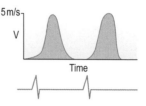

Peak velocity (V) of 5 m/s suggests a high pressure gradient ($4V^2 = 100$ mmHg) consistent with a restrictive VSD

Figure 6.11 Continuous wave Doppler showing high-velocity flow across a ventricular septal defect from left to right ventricle.

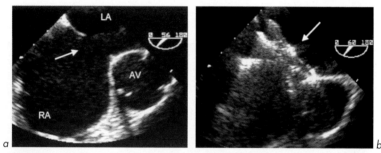

Figure 6.12 **(a)** Ostium secundum atrial septal defect (arrow). **(b)** Following percutaneous closure with Amplatzer device (arrow). Note the acoustic shadow cast by the device and seen in the right atrium on TOE.

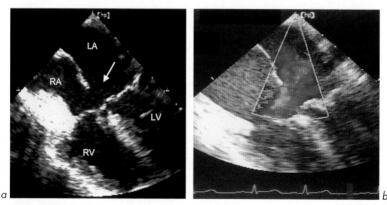

Figure 6.13 **(a)** Ostium primum atrial septal defect (arrow) on TOE 4-chamber view. **(b)** Colour flow mapping demonstrating flow across the defect.

Most clinically and haemodynamically significant ASDs should be diagnosed by TTE. However, TOE should be considered where left-to-right shunting is suspected but not confirmed on TTE (even after contrast study) or where a small defect may be significant (e.g. after trans-septal puncture at catheterization). TOE is superior at identifying associated abnormalities (e.g. partial anomalous pulmonary venous drainage).

PFO is seen in up to 30% at autopsy. TTE and TOE contrast studies show a prevalence of 10–35%. TOE colour flow mapping detects only one-third of those shown on contrast injection – for this reason, a contrast study should always be performed if a shunt is suspected.

Device closure for PFO may be considered in individuals who:
• Have suffered a stroke thought to be due to paradoxical (right-to-left) embolization across the PFO
• Suffer from migraine. Studies are still underway to determine whether this technique is an effective treatment in migraine.

Bubble/contrast studies (Fig. 6.14)

Contrast studies are often useful in determining whether there is flow across the interatrial septum (IAS) (see Section 5.3). This can be done with commercially available contrast agents or with saline which has a small amount of the patient's blood and air bubbles agitated in a syringe, to produce microbubbles. This is injected into a peripheral vein, and contrast is seen in the RA and then the RV. The subject is often asked to perform a Valsalva manoeuvre to increase intrathoracic pressure. Contrast may be seen shunting from RA to LA in the presence of an ASD or PFO, or RV to LV in the presence of a VSD. A bubble contrast study may be positive even when no obvious flow is detected on colour flow mapping.

Indications for bubble/contrast echo study include:
• Suspected PFO, ASD or VSD
• Dilated RA and/or dilated RV of unknown cause
• PHT of unknown cause.

In the investigation of a possible intracardiac shunt (caused, for example, by a PFO), a bubble contrast study may be considered positive if microbubbles are seen in the LA within 3–6 cardiac cycles after the appearance of the microbubbles in the RA. Ideally, microbubbles will be seen to cross the IAS through the PFO. Some grading schemes have been proposed, based upon the number and appearance of microbubbles and degree of opacification of the LA (e.g. no bubbles or mild, moderate or severe shunting). The appearance of microbubbles in the LA after 3–6 cardiac cycles usually indicates intrapulmonary shunting, such as an arteriovenous malformation. Intrapulmonary shunting is confirmed when the microbubbles are seen entering the LA from the pulmonary veins and not seen crossing

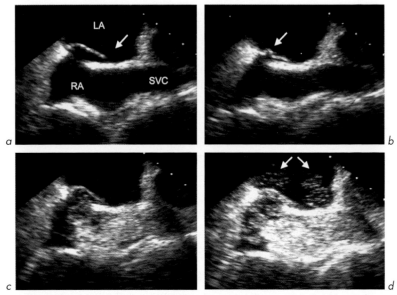

Figure 6.14 Patent foramen ovalve (PFO) and bubble contrast TOE study.
(a) The PFO is shown (arrow). **(b)** 'Buckling' of the interatrial septum (arrow).
(c) Bubble contrast reaches right atrium. **(d)** Some bubbles are seen to cross
the PFO from right to left atrium (arrows).

the IAS. Other causes for a false positive bubble study for PFO
are sinus venosus septal defect or other unidentified ASD or
'pseudocontrast' caused by the strain phase of the Valsalva manoeuvre,
with transient stagnation of blood in the pulmonary veins.

Causes of a false negative bubble contrast study:
- Inadequate opacification of the RA
- Inadequate Valsalva manoeuvre
- Inability to increase RA pressure above LA pressure, e.g. due to
  presence of LV diastolic dysfunction
- Poor echo image quality. The use of second-harmonic imaging can
  improve the identification and detection of microbubbles
- Eustachian valve, directing venous return from the IVC to the
  IAS, preventing microbubbles entering from the SVC to cross
  the IAS.

Patent ductus arteriosus

This is a condition in which the ductus arteriosus remains open after
birth. This provides a communication between the aorta and PA. A
continuous murmur occurs in systole and diastole (a 'machinery'
murmur). Echo can be used to detect the presence of the shunt and
give an estimate of its haemodynamic significance.

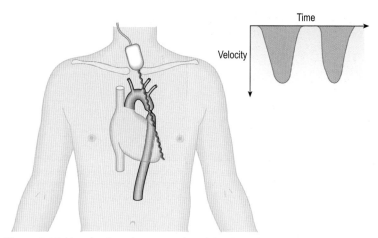

Figure 6.15 Examination of a coarctation of the thoracic aorta by continuous wave Doppler with the transducer in the suprasternal notch.

Eisenmenger reaction

This occurs when an intracardiac or extracardiac shunt is associated with PHT. Echo is very important in providing non-invasive assessment allowing the underlying cause to be seen (e.g. VSD), estimating the PASP by the peak Doppler velocity of TR and assessing complications such as severity of TR and size and function of the RV.

2. COARCTATION OF THE AORTA

Coarctation (narrowing) of the aorta may be detected using echo and the peak velocity across the coarctation (and hence the pressure gradient) can be measured. This is usually achieved using continuous wave Doppler with the transducer in the suprasternal notch (Figs. 1.11, 6.15).

3. CONGENITAL VALVULAR ABNORMALITIES

Bicuspid aortic valve (Fig. 6.16)

This is the most common congenital cardiac abnormality (1–2% of the population). This can be seen by its features on M-mode echo (eccentric closure line) and on 2-D echo, particularly in parasternal short-axis view at aortic level. It may occur in isolation or in association with other congenital conditions (e.g. coarctation). It may cause AS. Other abnormalities of the AV may be detected (e.g. 4-leaflet valve – very rare! [Fig. 6.17]).

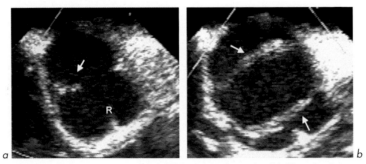

Figure 6.16 Bicuspid aortic valve – TOE short-axis study. **(a)** Closed valve showing eccentric closure line (arrow) and median raphe (R) representing the region where 2 leaflets are congenitally fused. **(b)** Open valve showing 2 leaflets (arrows).

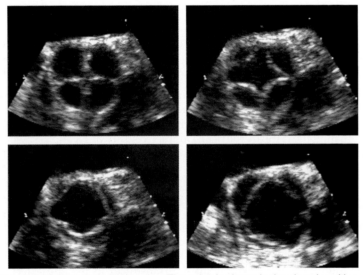

Figure 6.17 Four-cusp aortic valve. The valve is shown in the closed position and at various stages of opening. The anatomy was confirmed at surgery for severe aortic regurgitation. This congenital abnormality is very rare.

Ebstein's anomaly (Figs. 6.18, 6.19)

A rare but important group of abnormalities. The characteristic feature of this is TV dysplasia (malformation) with downward (apical) displacement of the TV into the body of the RV. There is consequent 'atrialization' of the upper part of the RV. Abnormalities of the TV leaflets and chordae include tricuspid atresia (absent development), and can cause TS or TR. 2-D and Doppler echo can show the abnormality present and its consequences.

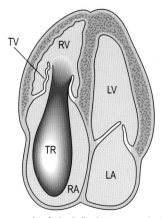

Figure 6.18 Ebstein's anomaly. Apical displacement of tricuspid valve (TV), which is often malformed causing tricuspid stenosis or severe regurgitation as shown.

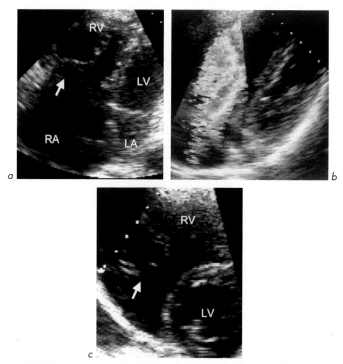

Figure 6.19 Ebstein's anomaly. **(a)** Apical 4-chamber view showing malformation of the tricuspid valve (arrow). **(b)** Colour flow mapping showing severe tricuspid regurgitation. **(c)** Parasternal short-axis view showing dilated right ventricle and malformed tricuspid valve (arrow).

Pulmonary stenosis

This may occur as a congenital abnormality and even quite high degrees of obstruction can be tolerated into adult life (particularly if RV function is good, there is no associated severe TR and sinus rhythm is maintained). It may be valvular or due to narrowing in the PA or RV outflow tract. Continuous wave Doppler and 2-D echo can assess severity, the effect upon RV size and function, associated congenital lesions and the presence and severity of TR.

4. CONGENITAL ATRIAL ABNORMALITIES

Cor triatriatum ('three-atrium heart') is a defect where the LA (or, much less often, RA) is subdivided by an additional membrane (septum). This may be fenestrated (with hole/s) or complete, giving the appearance of 3 atria. It represents 0.1% of all congenital cardiac abnormalities, but 50% of cases are associated with other cardiac defects, which determine the presentation (e.g. tetralogy of Fallot, double outlet RV, aortic coarctation, VSD). It may present at birth or in infancy with heart failure. The membrane can be surgically removed. It may be an incidental echo finding in adults (Fig. 6.20).

5. COMPLEX CONGENITAL ABNORMALITIES

These are beyond the scope of this book, but one condition is worth mentioning: **tetralogy of Fallot** (Figs. 6.21, 6.22) – characterized by:
1. VSD – usually perimembranous
2. Over-riding aorta – displaced to the right and loss of continuity with IVS
3. RV outflow tract obstruction (RVOTO) – at different sites, often in combination – infundibular (subvalvular) in 70–80%, valvular in 20–40%. Supravalvular is less common
4. RV hypertrophy.

Echo can help in diagnosis of tetralogy of Fallot, nowadays usually in infancy, and in follow-up after surgical repair to examine adequacy of VSD closure, residual RVOTO, severity of PR, and RV thickness and function.

6. ECHO METHOD TO ESTIMATE CARDIAC OUTPUT AND SHUNT SIZE

Echo can give an estimate of the size of a shunt (e.g. due to flow across an ASD or VSD). The method is simple but requires some

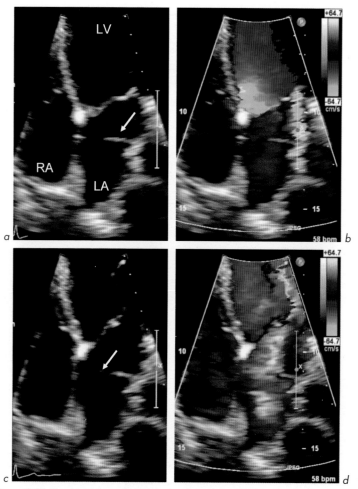

Figure 6.20 Cor triatriatum. Apical 4-chamber views. **(a)** Membrane subdividing left atrium (arrow). **(b)** Colour flow image when mitral valve closed. **(c)** Defect in membrane (arrow). **(d)** Colour flow through defect in membrane and from left atrium across open mitral valve to left ventricle. (Note there is no defect in the interatrial septum. The appearance is due to 'echo drop-out'.)

explanation. Using the continuity equation, the echo method to estimate cardiac output from the left heart was described in Chapter 3. This allows measurement of aortic or systemic flow (Qs). Now a similar method is applied also to the right heart. This allows measurement of pulmonary flow (Qp). The size of a shunt in an ASD or VSD can be estimated from the ratio of the pulmonary to the aortic flow. This ratio is Qp/Qs.

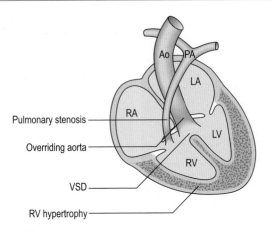

Figure 6.21 Tetralogy of Fallot.

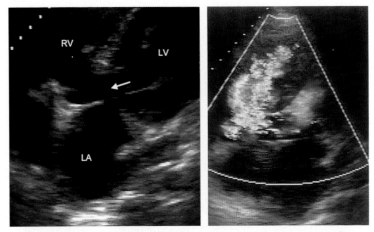

Figure 6.22 Tetralogy of Fallot. Colour flow through the ventricular septal defect (arrow) on apical 4-chamber view.

As a rough guide, a shunt is haemodynamically significant if the shunt ratio (Qp/Qs) is >2.0.

Figure 6.23 shows the method used.

Calculation of shunt size (Qp/Qs):

- For shunts due to ASDs or VSDs, the ratio Qp/Qs is the same as the ratio of stroke volume across the PV into the pulmonary circulation (SVp) to stroke volume across the AV into the systemic circulation (SVs) – i.e.

$$Qp/Qs = SVp/SVs$$

This is because the heart rate is the same for the left heart and the right heart.

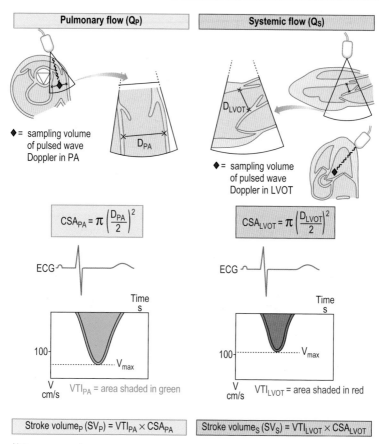

Figure 6.23 Echo method to calculate shunt size by measurement of systemic and pulmonary flow.

- Aortic flow, SVs (which equals flow across the LVOT) is given by:

$$SVs = CSA_{LVOT} \times VTI_{LVOT}$$

Where CSA_{LVOT} is the cross-sectional area of the LVOT and VTI_{LVOT} is the velocity time integral measured at the LVOT.

- Pulmonary flow, SVp, is given by:

$$SVp = CSA_{PA} \times VTI_{PA}$$

Where CSA_{PA} is the cross-sectional area of the PA and VTI_{PA} is the velocity time integral measured at the PA.

- The shunt ratio equation (Qp/Qs) simplifies to:

$$\frac{Q_P}{Q_s} = \frac{SV_P}{SV_s} = \frac{VTI_{PA} \times D_{PA}^2}{VTI_{LVOT} \times D_{LVOT}^2}$$

  - VTI_{PA} is usually measured from the Doppler signal of PA systolic flow from the parasternal short-axis view at aortic level
  - D_{PA} is the PA diameter in the same view
  - VTI_{LVOT} is usually measured at the LVOT using pulsed wave Doppler in the apical 5-chamber or long-axis views
  - D_{LVOT} is the diameter of the LVOT in the same views or parasternal long-axis view.

6.5 AORTA

The aorta is the largest artery in the body (Fig. 6.24) and carries oxygenated blood from the LV. The aorta is divided into:

- Aortic root (AV annulus, leaflets, sinuses of Valsalva and sinotubular junction) (Fig. 2.13)
- Ascending
- Arch
- Descending.

As with other arteries, the wall has 3 layers – intima, media and adventitia (Fig. 6.24).

IMPORTANCE OF AORTIC ROOT AND ASCENDING AORTA MEASUREMENTS

Echo can be used to examine the aorta. In adults, the first few centimetres of the aorta can be seen as a thin, echo-bright tube on TTE in parasternal long-axis and apical 5-chamber views (Figs. 1.3, 1.4, 1.13, 1.16, 1.18, 2.19). Echo (either M-mode or 2-D) can be used to measure the dimensions of the aortic root and ascending aorta at 4 points during end-diastole (apart from aortic annulus which is measured at mid-systole): AV annulus, sinuses of Valsalva, sinotubular junction and the ascending aorta (Fig. 2.13). The maximum diameters are in Table 6.2.

Detailed knowledge and quantification of aortic root and AV morphology is needed prior to AV surgery. It is also important with the increasing use of transcatheter AV implantation/replacement (TAVI/TAVR) procedures (see below).

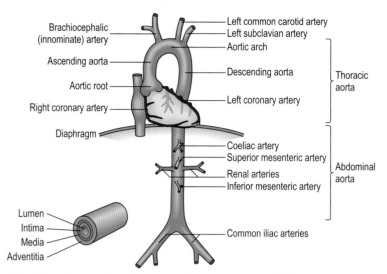

Figure 6.24 Aorta and main branches. Layers of aortic wall (inset).

Table 6.2 Echo measurements of aortic root and ascending aorta dimensions – normal values (cm)

	Women	Men
Aortic annulus	2.1–2.5	2.3–2.9
Sinuses of Valsalva	2.7–3.3	3.1–3.7
Sinotubular junction	2.3–2.9	2.6–3.2
Ascending aorta	2.3–3.1	2.6–3.4

Echo can be used to examine the aortic arch and its branches and ascending aorta, in TTE suprasternal and right parasternal views, respectively. These echo views may be difficult in adults. TOE (Chapter 5) gives excellent views of the ascending aorta, arch and descending aorta.

Aortic diseases include congenital abnormalities, such as coarctation (Section 6.4) and acquired conditions. These include atherosclerosis (which may be visualized on TTE, but particularly well with TOE), aortic aneurysm and aortic dissection (Section 5.1).

AORTIC ANEURYSM

An aneurysm is a fixed, localized dilatation of the aorta, diameter >50% of the upper limit of normal. It can occur in the ascending aorta, arch or descending aorta. A true aneurysm has all layers of the artery present. Aneurysms may be fusiform (symmetrical) or saccular (asymmetrical, with a narrow neck). The causes of, and risk factors for, aortic aneurysms are detailed in Figure 6.25.

Thoracic aorta

1 Weakened aortic wall
- atherosclerosis
- ageing (more common in people >65 years)
- tobacco smoking
- collagen and elastin disorders* – Marfan's, Ehlers-Danlos, pseudoxanthoma elasticum
- inflammation (aortitis) – ankylosing spondylitis, giant cell arteritis, Takayasu's, relapsing polychondritis
- infection – syphilis, TB, Salmonella
- post-trauma – deceleration injury, iatrogenic (e.g. post-cardiac catheter)
- familial (autosomal dominant)

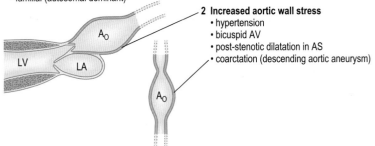

2 Increased aortic wall stress
- hypertension
- bicuspid AV
- post-stenotic dilatation in AS
- coarctation (descending aortic aneurysm)

Abdominal aorta

- tobacco smoking (>90%)
- atherosclerosis
- hypertension
- ageing
- genetic factors – esp. in males (4–6× increased risk in male siblings of affected individuals)
- collagen and elastin disorders causing cystic media necrosis (see * above)

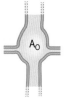

Figure 6.25 Aortic aneurysm. Causes and risk factors (these are similar for aortic dissection).

TTE may show aneurysms of the ascending aorta (Fig. 2.19) and aortic arch. TOE is an excellent technique to assess aneurysms throughout the aorta (Figs. 5.9, 7.2). The effects of aortic aneurysms depend upon their size and location. They may rupture (increased risk with increased diameter), cause pressure effects (e.g. on oesophagus, causing dysphagia) or be associated with other abnormalities (e.g. AR in Marfan's syndrome, Fig. 7.2). The decision whether surgically to treat an aortic aneurysm is based upon location, dimensions, effects, and co-existent cardiovascular and medical conditions. Abdominal aortic aneurysms (Fig. 6.25) can be assessed by ultrasound from the anterior abdominal wall.

AORTIC DISSECTION

This is a medical emergency and occurs when the intima shears away from the rest of the aortic wall, causing a dissection flap. Blood tracks along this plane and causes a false lumen and may re-enter the aorta further down (entry and exit points).

The causes of, and risk factors for, aortic dissection are similar to those of aortic aneurysms (Fig. 6.25). The location of the dissection determines the clinical presentation and treatment, which may be medical (the usual first line for dissections in the distal aorta) or surgical (the usual treatment for dissection of the proximal aorta – ascending and arch). Some cases of dissection in the descending aorta may be treated surgically or with aortic stenting. Clinical presentation of aortic dissection is usually with severe chest pain, often felt as a tearing sensation between the shoulder blades, or with the effects of the consequences of the dissection (e.g. acute heart failure due to acute AR, if the dissection involves the aortic root and AV). Figure 6.26 shows classifications of aortic dissection and treatments.

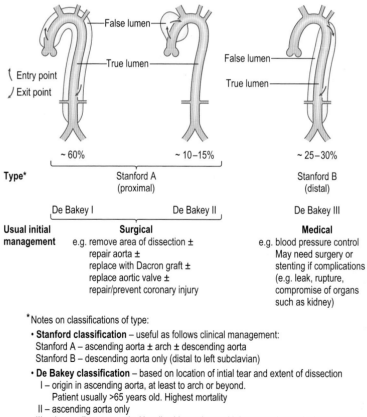

Type*	Stanford A (proximal)	Stanford B (distal)
	~ 60% ~ 10–15%	~ 25–30%
	De Bakey I De Bakey II	De Bakey III
Usual initial management	**Surgical** e.g. remove area of dissection ± repair aorta ± replace with Dacron graft ± replace aortic valve ± repair/prevent coronary injury	**Medical** e.g. blood pressure control May need surgery or stenting if complications (e.g. leak, rupture, compromise of organs such as kidney)

*Notes on classifications of type:
- **Stanford classification** – useful as follows clinical management:
  Stanford A – ascending aorta ± arch ± descending aorta
  Stanford B – descending aorta only (distal to left subclavian)
- **De Bakey classification** – based on location of intial tear and extent of dissection
  I – origin in ascending aorta, at least to arch or beyond.
     Patient usually >65 years old. Highest mortality
  II – ascending aorta only
  III – descending aorta only. Usually older patients with hypertension and atherosclerosis

Figure 6.26 Aortic dissection. Classifications and treatment.

TTE may show dissection of the ascending aorta and possible complications, such as AR. TOE (2-D and 3-D) is excellent in the assessment of aortic dissection (Figs. 5.9, 7.2).

TRANSCATHETER PROCEDURES ON AV AND AORTIC ROOT – TAVI (ALSO CALLED TAVR, PAVR)

Transcatheter AV implantation or replacement (TAVI, also termed TAVR), or percutaneous AV replacement (PAVR) are new techniques, increasingly used for the treatment of severe valvular AS in symptomatic patients where surgical (open) AV replacement is not possible or appropriate, for example due to existing severe co-morbidities.

TAVI involves the implantation of a stented prosthetic AV across the native stenosed AV (Fig. 6.27). This is usually by a percutaneous catheter approach through the common femoral artery, although there are transapical, transaortic and transcaval approaches. The native AV is held open by the stented valve. The procedure can also be performed in cases of stenotic prosthetic tissue AV replacements (Fig. 6.28).

Echo plays a vital role at every stage of these new procedures. Many echo modalities are of use: 2-D and 3-D echo, TTE and TOE. Echo is useful in:

- Pre-procedure preparation – assessing the severity of AS, measuring annular dimensions to select the correct size of stented AV (either by TTE or TOE, 2-D or 3-D), assessing if AV is tri-leaflet or bi-leaflet (technically more difficult), root and LVOT anatomy.

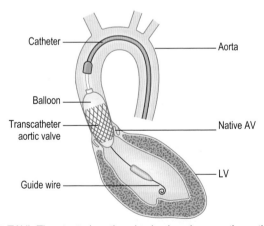

Catheter — Aorta

Balloon

Transcatheter aortic valve — Native AV

LV

Guide wire

Figure 6.27 TAVI. The stented aortic valve is placed across the native stenosed aortic valve, which remains open. After implantation, the balloon is deflated and removed with the guidewire and catheter.

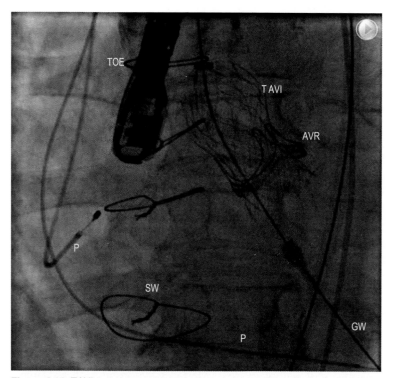

Figure 6.28 TAVI to treat a patient who has a stenosed prosthetic tissue aortic valve. Chest radiograph during the procedure shows TAVI, prosthetic aortic valve (AVR), TOE probe (TOE), pacing wire (P), guidewire (GW), sternal wires (SW) from previous median sternotomy for AV replacement.

Assessment of LV function. Assessment of PA systolic pressure. Assessment of co-existent valve lesions (e.g. MR and intracardiac thrombus). Other imaging modalities (such as CT and cardiac MRI) may also be helpful, for example, in identifying the origins of the coronary arteries and their relation to the AV annulus

- Intra-procedure monitoring – using TOE. This is not always used and requires general anaesthesia. It may be useful in some cases, especially during the procedural learning stages. It can help with correct placement of the prosthesis (in conjunction with X-ray fluoroscopy) (Fig. 6.28).
- Immediate post-procedure assessment for complications and success
- Late post-procedure assessment – follow-up adequacy of procedure (e.g. assessment of any AR), assessment of LV function and PA systolic pressure.

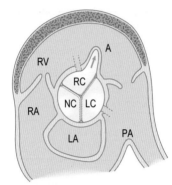

Figure 6.29 Sinus of Valsalva aneurysm. Parasternal short-axis view at right ventricular outflow (AV) level. The aneurysm (A, arrow) is shown arising in the right coronary (RC) sinus and protruding into the RV. This is the most frequent location. The left coronary (LC) and non-coronary (NC) sinuses are shown. The coronary artery origins are shown as dashed lines.

SINUS OF VALSALVA ANEURYSM

The sinuses of Valsalva are outpouchings of the aorta, from which the coronary arteries arise (Fig. 2.13). These may become aneurysmally dilated for several reasons:

• Congenital (associated with VSD)
• Aortic root pathology (e.g. Marfan's syndrome, Ehlers-Danlos, infection such as infective endocarditis or syphilis)
• Iatrogenic – following cardiac catheterization or surgery.

Sinus of Valsalva aneurysms protrude into adjacent chambers (right coronary sinus into RV in 65–85%, non-coronary sinus into RA in 10–30%, left coronary sinus into LA in <5%) (Fig. 6.29). Although often asymptomatic, they may rupture, causing a fistula and an abnormal shunt (e.g. aorta to RV) and may then require surgery.

SPECIAL SITUATIONS AND CONDITIONS

7.1 PREGNANCY

Echo in pregnancy is safe. Many pregnant women develop systolic murmurs due to increased cardiac output (which rises by 30–50% in pregnancy). Many murmurs are benign (e.g. mammary souffle) but some may not be. Cardiac disease can present and be diagnosed for the first time during pregnancy, or women with pre-existing heart disease may become pregnant and may experience deterioration in their cardiac state. Echo is essential in both situations. Some may experience troublesome palpitations and whilst this is a less clear-cut indication for echo, the finding of normal LV function, chamber size and valve function can be very reassuring.

Anatomical and echo changes in pregnancy can include:
- Mild increases in cardiac chamber size including RA and RV. LA increases by 10–15% and LV by 5–10%
- Increased stroke volume (increased velocity time integral of AV and PV)
- Small pericardial effusions (20%) causing no haemodynamic compromise. If there is compromise, another cause must be sought
- Peripartum cardiomyopathy
- Vascular 'laxity' in peripartum period. Both aortic and coronary artery spontaneous dissections are more common, but still rare
- In late pregnancy, the enlarged uterus may increase intra-abdominal pressure causing compression of the thoracic structures and a pseudo-posterior wall motion abnormality, as occurs in liver disease with ascites.

Of course, there are a number of congenital cardiac abnormalities that have important implications for pregnancy.

The body of knowledge relating to high cardiac-risk pregnancies is increasing. Many women with such pregnancies are managed in specialized centres where a multi-disciplinary team including obstetricians, midwives, cardiologists, anaesthetists, cardiac physiologists and nurses work together to minimize the risks. Echo often plays an important part in the decision-making process.

1. CARDIAC LESIONS ASSOCIATED WITH HIGH RISK (TO MOTHER)

- PHT (primary or secondary to Eisenmenger)
- Severe AS
- Severe MS
- Marfan's syndrome
- HOCM (especially if high degree of outflow tract obstruction)
- Any lesion causing NYHA Grade IV breathlessness (i.e. at rest or on minimal exertion)
- Some complex cardiac abnormalities (details below).

Eisenmenger's reaction (PHT with a shunt) carries a high maternal (30–70%) and fetal mortality. Maternal mortality is due to arrhythmia, increased cyanosis, low cardiac output, catastrophic rise in PA pressure and right heart failure. The early postpartum period is particularly dangerous, possibly related to sudden alterations in venous return.

In AS or MS, pregnancy increases the valve gradient as cardiac output rises and systemic vascular resistance falls. MS can be very difficult in pregnancy. Echo allows non-invasive assessment of the valve orifice and PA pressures and may help to determine timing of delivery or valvotomy.

In Marfan's syndrome, the dominant hazard is aortic root dilatation and aortic dissection, made more likely by haemodynamic changes and weakening of the aortic wall by hormonal changes.

Echo allows serial non-invasive assessment of PASP during pregnancy when this is elevated (e.g. primary or secondary to MV disease or Eisenmenger's).

2. INTERMEDIATE (MODERATE) RISK LESIONS

- Coarctation
- Cyanotic heart disease without PHT
- Prosthetic valves – risks are of premature valve failure (biological prostheses), thromboembolism, complications related to warfarin/heparin (e.g. teratogenesis, fetal growth retardation, placental haemorrhage, osteoporosis)
- Tetralogy of Fallot – can behave unpredictably – increased venous return and systemic vasodilatation can cause profound hypoxia.
- HCM.

3. LOWER-RISK LESIONS ARE FORTUNATELY THE MOST COMMON

* Uncomplicated ASD or VSD, although there is a risk of paradoxical embolization. One particular problem of unoperated ASD or VSD occurs at delivery. Blood loss may lower RA pressure and increase left-to-right shunting, stealing from the systemic circulation, sometimes progressively and catastrophically. Intravenous fluid replacement must be rigorous in these patients
* MR, AR and PS are usually well tolerated in pregnancy.

A detailed classification of maternal risk during pregnancy, based upon the underlying cardiac condition, is summarized in Tables 7.1 and 7.2.

Benign maternal murmurs in pregnancy (see Section 1.6)

* Pulmonary flow murmur – at left sternal edge at 2nd intercostal space. Due to increased cardiac output and flow into the pulmonary circulation
* Venous hum
* Mammary souffle – associated with lactation and ceasing when that ends.

Table 7.1 Modified WHO classification of maternal cardiovascular risk in pregnancy – risk classes

Risk class	Risk of pregnancy due to medical condition
I	• No detectable increased risk of maternal mortality, and • No/mild increased risk of maternal morbidity
II	• Small increased risk of maternal mortality, or • Moderately increased risk of maternal morbidity
III	• Significantly increased risk of maternal mortality, or • Severely increased risk of maternal morbidity *Expert counselling needed. If decision is for pregnancy, intensive specialist obstetric and cardiac monitoring throughout pregnancy, childbirth and puerperium.*
IV	• Extremely high risk of maternal mortality, or • Severely increased maternal morbidity *Pregnancy contraindicated. If pregnancy occurs, termination should be discussed. If pregnancy continues, care as for Class III.*

Adapted from Thorne S, MacGregor A, Nelson-Piercy C. Risks of contraception and pregnancy in heart disease. Heart 2006;92:1520–1525 and Regitz-Zagrosek V, Blomstrom Lundqvist C, Borghi C, et al. ESC Guidelines on the management of cardiovascular diseases during pregnancy: the Task Force on the Management of Cardiovascular Diseases during Pregnancy of the European Society of Cardiology (ESC). Eur Heart J. 2011;32:3147–197.
WHO, World Health Organization.

Table 7.2 Modified World Health Organization (WHO) classification of maternal cardiovascular risk in pregnancy – cardiac conditions

Cardiac conditions in which pregnancy risk is WHO I:
- Uncomplicated, small or mild:
  - PS
  - MV prolapse
  - PDA
- Successfully repaired simple lesions:
  - ASD
  - VSD
  - PDA
  - anomalous pulmonary venous drainage
- Atrial or ventricular ectopic beats, isolated

Cardiac conditions in which pregnancy risk is WHO II or III:

WHO II (if otherwise well and uncomplicated)
- Unoperated ASD
- Unoperated VSD
- Repaired tetralogy of Fallot
- Most arrhythmias

WHO II or III (depending on individual)
- Mild LV impairment
- HCM
- Native or tissue valvular heart disease not considered WHO I or IV
- Marfan's syndrome without aortic dilatation
- Aorta <45 mm in aortic disease associated with bicuspid AV
- Repaired aortic coarctation

WHO III
- Mechanical valve
- Systemic RV
- Fontan circulation
- Cyanotic heart disease (unrepaired)
- Other complex congenital heart disease
- Aortic dilatation 40–45 mm in Marfan's syndrome
- Aortic dilatation 45–50 mm in aortic disease associated with bicuspid AV

Cardiac conditions in which pregnancy risk is WHO IV (pregnancy contraindicated):
- Pulmonary arterial hypertension of any cause
- Severe systemic ventricular dysfunction (LVEF <30%, NYHA III–IV)
- Previous peripartum cardiomyopathy with any residual impairment of LV function
- Severe MS
- Severe symptomatic AS
- HOCM with severe LVOTO
- Marfan's syndrome with aorta dilated >45 mm
- Aortic dilatation >50 mm in aortic disease associated with bicuspid AV
- Native severe aortic coarctation

Adapted from Thorne S, MacGregor A, Nelson-Piercy C. Risks of contraception and pregnancy in heart disease. Heart *2006;92:1520–1525 and Regitz-Zagrosek V, Blomstrom Lundqvist C, Borghi C, et al. ESC Guidelines on the management of cardiovascular diseases during pregnancy: the Task Force on the Management of Cardiovascular Diseases during Pregnancy of the European Society of Cardiology (ESC).* Eur Heart J. *2011;32:3147–3197.*

Peripartum cardiomyopathy

Echo shows a dilated LV with impaired systolic function. It presents in the later part of pregnancy and in the postpartum months. The echo features are identical to those of dilated cardiomyopathy. It may represent pre-existing dilated cardiomyopathy undiagnosed before pregnancy. The prognosis relates to the severity of heart failure and how rapidly cardiac size returns to normal. If present for more than 6 months, the prognosis is poor. Treatment is conventional (diuretics and ACE inhibitors). It may recur in subsequent pregnancies.

Fetal welfare

The risks mentioned relate to the mother. Fetal welfare must of course be assessed during these pregnancies. The hazards to the fetus relate to:

1. Maternal cyanosis
2. Need for bypass surgery during pregnancy (20% risk of fetal loss)
3. Drug therapy:
   - Warfarin – fetal haemorrhage and multiple congenital abnormalities
   - Heparin – retroplacental haemorrhage
   - ACE inhibitors – neonatal renal failure, oligohydramnios, growth retardation
   - β-Blockers – intrauterine growth restriction, neonatal hypoglycaemia, bradycardia
4. Genetic risk of transmission
   - Marfan's syndrome, HCM and other single gene defects – 50%
   - Multi-factorial conditions such as ASD or VSD – transmission rate 4–6%, compared with prevalence in the general population of 1%.

Fetal echo

Fetal echo (by transabdominal or transvaginal ultrasound examination) is carried out in a number of specialist centres to determine if there is a cardiac abnormality in the unborn child. Some cases have been surgically corrected *in utero*.

7.2 RHYTHM DISTURBANCES

Arrhythmias can be primary abnormalities or occur in association with structural heart disease. This may include congenital abnormalities or those of the myocardium, valves, pericardium or coronary arteries. The main use of echo is in determining associated heart disease.

ATRIAL FIBRILLATION (AF) OR FLUTTER

Fibrillation refers to the situation when electrical activity is not co-ordinated in a chamber and individual muscle fibres contract independently. This can occur in atrial or ventricular muscle. Ventricular fibrillation (VF), unless promptly terminated, is fatal. AF can be tolerated, and, apart from the occurrence of atrial and ventricular extrasystoles, is the most common arrhythmia in many countries. An underlying cause for AF should always be sought.

Common causes of AF
• Ischaemic heart disease
• Rheumatic heart disease (e.g. MS)
• Hypertension
• Toxins (e.g. ethanol)
• Thyroid disease – usually thyrotoxicosis
• Infection – myocarditis, pneumonia
• Myocardial disease (e.g. dilated cardiomyopathy)
• Lung disease
• Pulmonary embolism
• Pericardial disease (e.g. pericarditis)
• 'Lone' – no underlying cause found.

All individuals with AF should have an echo. This is to determine an underlying cause (e.g. MS), assess the risk of complications (such as stroke, see below) and assess the likelihood of successful restoration to normal sinus rhythm (cardioversion) by electrical or chemical means.

Echo detects an underlying cardiac disorder in approximately 10% of people with AF who have no other clinically suspected heart disease and in 60% of people with some indicators of heart disease.

AF can be classified as:
• Acute – onset within 48 hours
• Paroxysmal – spontaneous termination (return to sinus rhythm), usually within 48 hours (or up to 7 days)
• Recurrent – 2 or more episodes – paroxysmal, if self-terminating, or persistent, if AF requires electrical or pharmacological cardioversion. May require pharmacological or catheter ablation treatment for symptom control
• Persistent – not self-terminating, lasting more than 7 days
• Permanent – lasting more than 1 year (e.g. not treated successfully with cardioversion). Return to sinus rhythm may be possible, especially after treatment of an underlying cause of AF (e.g. thyrotoxicosis) or with catheter ablation.

Restoration of sinus rhythm is *less* likely to be successful if there is:
- MV disease
- An enlarged LA
- LV dysfunction
- Thyroid disease
- Long-standing AF.

Unless there is a contraindication, individuals with AF have an improved prognosis if treated with anticoagulants such as warfarin. This is certainly true for rheumatic AF and probably in non-rheumatic AF where there is an underlying cause. It is less certain in 'lone' AF. This benefit increases with the age of the individual.

The annual risk of stroke is increased in subjects with LA enlargement or LV dysfunction (Table 7.3).

There is evidence to suggest that, in many people with AF, heart rate control (e.g. with digoxin, β-blockers or calcium-channel blockers) and long-term anticoagulation with warfarin is preferable to attempting rhythm control (i.e. cardioversion). Cardioversion may be considered if:
- Recent-onset AF with an identifiable reversible cause (e.g. recent treated pneumonia)
- Subject is very symptomatic and unable to tolerate AF and/or rate-controlling medications
- AF has caused heart failure
- Individual is unable to take long-term anticoagulants.

Following successful cardioversion, warfarin should be continued for 3–6 months, since the return of atrial mechanical activity (at which time thromboembolism might occur) is often delayed, due to atrial

Table 7.3 Annual stroke risk for different cardiac parameters

Findings	Annual stroke risk (%)
Normal heart – sinus rhythm	0.3
'Lone' AF	0.5
AF with normal echo	1.5
AF with enlarged LA >2.5 cm/m^2	8.8
AF with global LV dysfunction	12.6
AF with enlarged LA (>2.5 cm/m^2) and moderate LV dysfunction	20.0

Data from Stroke Prevention in Atrial Fibrillation Study Group Investigators. Predictors of thromboembolism in atrial fibrillation: II. Echocardiographic features of patients at risk. The Stroke Prevention in Atrial Fibrillation Investigators. Ann Intern Med. 1992;116:6–12.

'stunning', relative to the restoration of synchronized atrial electrical activity.

There are newer (novel) oral anticoagulants (NOACs – e.g. dabigatran, rivaroxaban, apixaban), which are suitable as an alternative to warfarin in appropriate patients with AF (e.g. non-rheumatic AF).

In some patients with AF, catheter ablation of the rhythm disturbance is considered, particularly in those with troublesome symptoms and/or intolerance of anti-arrhythmic drugs. Sometimes, more than one ablation procedure is necessary. In people with a structurally normal heart, success rates for catheter ablation are:
- Recurrent (paroxysmal) AF: ~70–75% (1st ablation), >90% (with 2 ablations)
- Persistent AF: ~60% (1st ablation), ~80% (with 2 ablations).

Echo before cardioversion

This may help to identify patients most likely to have successful cardioversion to sinus rhythm or to predict those at increased risk of thromboembolic complications. Previous data suggest that 5–7% of subjects undergoing cardioversion who have not been anticoagulated experience thromboembolic complications. These may not occur until some time after cardioversion. The most likely explanation is that atrial mechanical activity may not return for some time after the restoration of atrial electrical activity.

There is some controversy regarding the use of TOE in patients with persistent AF (>48 hours) prior to cardioversion. Pre- and post-cardioversion anticoagulation is indicated and large studies are underway. There is less information in recent-onset AF (<48 hours) but present data suggest that 14% of patients with recent AF have LA appendage thrombus, suggesting that these patients should also receive anticoagulation.

Indications for TOE before cardioversion

- Urgent cardioversion needed when pre-cardioversion anticoagulation not possible
- Prior thromboembolic events thought to be related to LA thrombus
- Previous demonstration of LA thrombus
- If finding co-existent factors influences decision to cardiovert (e.g. LV function, MV disease)
- AF of <48 hours
- AF in the presence of MV disease or HCM, even if anticoagulated.

VENTRICULAR TACHYCARDIA (VT) OR FIBRILLATION (VF)

These are important indications for echo. The underlying cause is often coronary artery disease, and there may be features of ischaemia and/or infarction. VT of LV origin is frequently associated with reduced LV function. It may complicate an underlying cardiomyopathy (e.g. dilated or hypertrophic). VT of RV origin may suggest an RV structural abnormality such as arrhythmogenic cardiomyopathy (AC; also referred to as arrhythmogenic RV cardiomyopathy or dysplasia, Section 4.4).

SYNCOPE

This means sudden loss of consciousness. It can have a number of neurological or cardiac causes. The role of echo relates to its ability to detect obstructive lesions (e.g. AS, HCM) or abnormalities such as LV impairment that may be associated with arrhythmias such as VT. The use of echo routinely in patients with syncope is controversial.

Indications include:

- Syncope with suspected heart disease
- Exertional syncope
- Syncope in high-risk occupation (e.g. pilot).

PALPITATIONS

Many people experience atrial or ventricular ectopic beats. The indication for echo in these cases is less clear-cut. An echo should be carried out if there is any suspicion of structural heart disease (abnormality on history, e.g. associated symptoms such as syncope, clinical examination, ECG or chest X-ray). Otherwise the pick-up rate is very low. A normal echo (normal LV, other chambers and valves) can be reassuring for an anxious individual.

In general, echo does not need to be performed in a person with palpitations for which an arrhythmic cause has been ruled out.

7.3 STROKE, TIA AND THROMBOEMBOLISM

'IS THERE A CARDIAC SOURCE OF EMBOLISM?'

This is a fairly common question asked when an echo is requested. It can be quite difficult to answer, particularly by TTE. TOE may provide more information.

Ultrasound examination of patients with stroke or TIA in territories outside the vertebrobasilar territories is certainly important but echo is not the only useful test. Ultrasound scanning of the carotid arteries may provide useful diagnostic information and finding significant carotid stenosis (>70%) is an indication for carotid endarterectomy.

In the presence of a normal cardiovascular history, examination and ECG, the likelihood of a TTE detecting a cardiac abnormality in stroke or TIA is very low.

The main purposes of echo are:

- To make a diagnosis associated with risk of thromboembolism (e.g. MS, LV dilatation)
- To detect a direct source of embolism from an intracardiac mass – thrombus, tumour, vegetation.

Indications for echo in stroke, TIA or vascular occlusive events

- Sudden occlusion of a peripheral or visceral artery
- Younger patients (<50 years) with stroke or TIA
- Older patients (>50 years) with stroke or TIA without evidence of cerebrovascular disease or other obvious cause
- Suspicion of embolic disease
- Clinical evidence of cardiac abnormality (e.g. abnormal physical signs (murmur, suspected endocarditis) or abnormal ECG (MI, arrhythmia such as AF, VT or non-specific ST-T abnormalities)).

TOE may be indicated (with a normal or inconclusive TTE) if:

- High suspicion of embolism (e.g. endocarditis)
- Young patient (many centres arbitrarily say age <50 years).

The risk of thromboembolism is so high in MS, particularly if AF is present, that anticoagulation should be considered if there is no contraindication and cerebral haemorrhage has been excluded by CT scanning. This is true even if the echo does not show obvious thrombus (remember, LA thrombus is often not seen on TTE). Alternatively, echo may show a large LA ball thrombus, which is an indication for urgent surgery (see Box 7.1).

In young people, it is generally agreed that TTE and TOE should be carried out to look for treatable rare causes of stroke such as:

- Left atrial myxoma (which has been estimated to occur in 1% of such cases)
- LA spontaneous contrast
- LA appendage thrombus
- PFO (venous thrombus can 'paradoxically' embolize from right to left)
- Aneurysm of IAS (increased risk of thromboembolism possibly due to frequent association with PFO)
- Aortic atheroma.

7.4 HYPERTENSION AND LVH (Fig. 7.1)

MAIN INDICATIONS FOR ECHO IN HYPERTENSION

- Assessment of LV systolic and diastolic function
- Detection of LVH and response to treatment
- Detection/effects of co-existing coronary disease (e.g. by stress echo)
- Possible underlying cause of hypertension (e.g. aortic coarctation).

> **Box 7.1** Echo in systemic embolization –
> underlying diagnoses and possible echo findings
> (TOE is most useful)
>
> - LA thrombus – usually in LA appendage. Best seen using TOE
> - LA spontaneous contrast
> - LV mural thrombus – LV thrombus, usually associated with regional akinesia or LV aneurysm
> - Atrial myxoma – mass attached to interatrial septum (IAS)
> - Infective endocarditis – vegetation
> - Paradoxical embolism – PFO and/or aneurysmal IAS
> - Papillary fibroelastoma – valvular mass
> - Aortic atheroma – in ascending, arch or descending aorta. Best seen using TOE
> - Prosthetic valve thrombus – Thrombus and/or valve dysfunction. Best seen using TOE

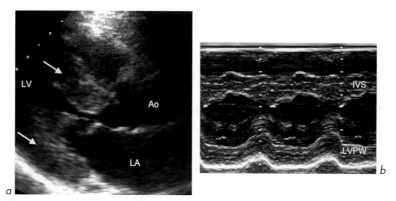

Figure 7.1 Severe concentric left ventricular hypertrophy (LVH) in long-standing hypertension. **(a)** Parasternal long-axis view showing LVH of septum and posterior wall (arrows). **(b)** M-mode.

Hypertension is the most important cause of LVH, which is an independent predictive factor for cardiovascular mortality and morbidity. It predicts the risk of MI, heart failure or sudden cardiac death and is as predictive as the occurrence of multi-vessel coronary artery disease. LVH may be indicated on voltage criteria on ECG recording (large voltage QRS complexes). The criteria differ but S in V1 or V2 plus R in V5 or V6 >35 mm is useful (Sokolow-Lyon criteria). Some patients with thin chest walls may have voltage criteria for LVH on ECG but normal LV wall thickness. There may be associated 'strain pattern' on ECG in LVH (ST segment depression and T-wave inversion in the lateral leads).

Echo allows wall thickness to be measured accurately and is more sensitive than ECG at detecting LVH. The presence of LVH can help to determine if treatment is necessary in people with borderline hypertension. Echo can also be used to assess whether there is regression of LVH with antihypertensive treatment.

ECHO TECHNIQUES TO ESTIMATE LV MASS

LVH is often considered present if the IVS or LVPW thickness is above 'normal limits' (often >12 mm in diastole). Strictly speaking, one should measure LV mass to diagnose LVH.

LV mass can be calculated from echo using several techniques, based upon different geometrical models of the LV:

- Linear method – measurements using M-mode echo (or 2-D echo) using the cubed formula below
- 2-D methods using the area–length formula or truncated ellipsoid formula
- 3-D echo.

The linear method (cubed formula), which incorporates only one dimension of the LV cavity and assumes an ellipsoid geometry, is the most widely used to calculate LV volumes and LV mass. M-mode echo estimation was the first method to be validated and also has technical simplicity. The one-dimensional approach, however, imposes more strict geometrical assumptions and amplifies the risk of inaccuracy, as measurement errors are cubed.

The cubed formula for LV mass uses linear M-mode (or 2-D) measurements of IVS and LVPW thickness in diastole and LVEDD, all in cm, by an equation initially suggested by Troy et al. (*Circulation* 1972; 45: 602–11), which was modified by Devereux et al. (*Am J Cardiol.* 1986; 57: 450–8):

$$LV\ mass\ (g) = 0.8 \times 1.04 \times [(LVEDD + IVS + LVPW)^3 - LVEDD^3] + 0.6$$

LV mass should be corrected for height or BSA (which gives 'LV mass index'). The 'normal values' using the linear method above (and for a 2-D method) are in Table 7.4.

As with other 'normal' echo ranges, characterization of the population being studied and differences in LV mass between different ethnic populations should be taken into account when determining normal values.

Advantages of linear method for estimating LV mass:

- Fast and widely used
- Wealth of published data

Table 7.4 Normal ranges for LV mass indices

	Women	Men
LV mass (g) – linear method (M-mode echo, cubed formula)	67–162	88–224
LV mass corrected for BSA ('LV mass index') (g/m²) – linear method	*43–95*	*49–115*
Septal thickness (cm) – diastole	*0.6–0.9*	*0.6–1.0*
Posterior wall thickness (cm) – diastole	*0.6–0.9*	*0.6–1.0*
LV mass – 2-D echo method	66–150	96–200
LV mass corrected for BSA ('LV mass index') (g/m²) – 2-D echo method	*44–88*	*50–102*

Bold italic values: recommended and best validated.
Based upon Lang RM, Badano LP, Mor-Avi V, et al. Recommendations for cardiac chamber quantification by echocardiography in adults: an update from the American Society of Echocardiography and the European Association of Cardiovascular Imaging. J Am Soc Echocardiogr. 2015;28:1–39.

- Demonstrated prognostic value
- Fairly accurate in normally shaped ventricles (e.g. AS, hypertension)
- Simple for screening large populations.

Limitations of linear method for estimating LV mass:
- Based on the assumption that LV is a prolate ellipsoid with a 2:1 long:short axis ratio and symmetrical distribution of hypertrophy
- Ultrasound beam frequently off-axis
- Since linear measurements are cubed, even small measurement errors in dimensions or thickness have an impact on accuracy
- Overestimates LV mass
- Inaccurate in the presence of asymmetric hypertrophy, dilated ventricles and other diseases with regional variations in wall thickness.

If a 2-D approach is used, both area–length and truncated–ellipsoid models are feasible and reasonably accurate, with validated formulas, but tend to be less well validated than linear methods and the values calculated by the 2-D methods are often lower than those by the linear method.

3-D echo techniques may allow direct measurement without geometrical assumptions about cavity shape and the distribution of hypertrophy. May be more accurate than the linear or the 2-D measurement. There are, as yet, no normal value data.

7.5 BREATHLESSNESS AND PERIPHERAL OEDEMA

Breathlessness is an important symptom of many heart diseases. In the presence of heart failure, it usually indicates pulmonary venous hypertension. The causes of breathlessness are numerous. Cardiac diseases often co-exist with respiratory causes such as chronic airflow limitation.

Echo is an essential test in a breathless patient where the history, examination and routine tests such as ECG and chest X-ray suggest or cannot exclude heart disease. It may reveal:
- LV systolic and/or diastolic dysfunction
- Left-sided valve disease
- Cardiomyopathy.

The use of echo in the assessment of people with acute severe breathlessness is discussed in Section 5.5.

Oedema has a number of cardiac and non-cardiac causes. The cardiac causes are any conditions that increase the central venous pressure and include myocardial, pericardial and valvular abnormalities. Echo is useful in these cases. In cases of peripheral oedema with a normal JVP, echo is *not* likely to be helpful (unless the patient has been receiving treatment with diuretics).

Other causes of oedema should be investigated:
- Renal failure
- Protein-losing states (e.g. nephrotic syndrome)
- Hypoalbuminaemia (e.g. liver disease)
- Deep venous thrombosis
- Venous incompetence
- Pelvic obstruction
- Endocrine abnormality (e.g. hypothyroidism).

7.6 SCREENING AND FOLLOW-UP ECHO

WHO SHOULD HAVE A SCREENING ECHO?

If screening asymptomatic individuals, some criteria should be met:
- The test should be safe, accurate, readily available and inexpensive – echo satisfies these
- The abnormality should have a reasonable frequency to allow detection
- Detection should alter management or provide prognostic information.

There are no clear-cut rules. Some suggestions:

Good indications for screening echo

1. Individuals with a family history of genetically transmitted cardiovascular disease:

- First-degree relatives of people with HCM – many screen every 5 years from age 5 up to age 20 (if normal by that age, the diagnosis is excluded). Approximately 1 in 5 first-degree relatives of people with HCM were found to have the condition in a large-scale screening study
  - Suspected collagen abnormalities (e.g. Marfan's syndrome [should correct values for body size and age], Ehlers–Danlos)
  - First-degree relatives of people with myxomas (some rare familial forms associated with multiple freckles and HCM) or tuberous sclerosis.
2. Potential cardiac transplantation donors (in ICU) by TTE or TOE. The overall yield for conditions that eliminate the heart as a donor is approximately 1 in 4.
3. Baseline and follow-up re-evaluations of patients with cancer undergoing chemotherapy with cardiotoxic agents (see Section 7.9).

Less clear-cut indications for screening echo

1. High risk of LV impairment
   - Post-MI
   - Alcohol excess
   - Hypertension with LVH
   - LBBB in a young patient.
2. Systemic diseases that may affect the heart (see Section 7.8).

'Follow-up' echo

This is performed in patients with some cardiac diseases at the intervals suggested below (more frequently if a clinical indication of deterioration such as development of new symptoms in previously controlled valve disease):
- Severe AS: 3–6 months
- Moderate AS: annual
- Moderate AR: 3–6 months
- HCM: annual
- Dilated aortic root: 6–12 months
- MV disease: annual
- Artificial biological valves: after 5 years then annual
- LV impairment: based on symptoms
- Following resection of cardiac tumour: annual for up to 5 years (recurrence rare).

7.7 ADVANCED AGE

There are predictable echo changes with advanced age:
- Progressive angulation between the descending aorta and the LVOT

- Localized proximal septal bulge resulting in a sigmoid shape to the proximal ventricular septum (upper septal bulge)
- Thickening of aortic wall
- Focal thickening of AV, MV and chordae
- MV annular calcification
- Increased myocardial stiffness causing diastolic function changes detected on pulsed wave Doppler as changes in the E:A ratio
- Mild LA dilatation
- A pattern mimicking HCM may develop, especially with hypertension that is poorly controlled.

7.8 ECHO ABNORMALITIES IN SOME SYSTEMIC DISEASES AND CONDITIONS

Some of these echo features may be present.

1. INFECTIONS

HIV infection and AIDS

- Dilated cardiomyopathy
- Myocarditis (e.g. due to opportunistic infections such as *Toxoplasma*, *Histoplasma*, cytomegalovirus)
- Pericardial effusion and tamponade
- Non-bacterial thrombotic endocarditis (marantic)
- Infective endocarditis (e.g. *Aspergillus*)
- Metastases from Kaposi's sarcoma
- PHT
- RV failure due to recurrent chest infections and PHT
- Effects of associated coronary disease.

Chagas' disease

This is caused by *Trypanosoma cruzi* and is endemic in Central and South America. It is one of the most common causes of heart failure worldwide with 20 million people affected.
- Myocarditis in acute stages
- Echo features similar to dilated cardiomyopathy
- Apical aneurysm common.

Lyme disease

This is caused by the tick-borne spirochaete *Borrelia burgdorferi*. It is characterized by erythema chronicum migrans and an acute systemic illness. The disease is endemic in many parts of the world. Untreated, late rheumatological, neurological and cardiac complications are frequent; the latter can include severe symptomatic high-degree atrioventricular block, which may necessitate permanent pacemaker implantation. Early treatment with antibiotics (such as tetracyclines or penicillins) may reduce complications.

* Myocarditis, pericarditis
* LV dysfunction.

2. INFLAMMATORY, RHEUMATIC AND CONNECTIVE TISSUE DISEASES

Marfan's syndrome (Fig. 7.2)

This is an autosomal dominant condition, so relatives must be screened (see Section 7.6). Spontaneous mutation may occur in up to 30% of patients.

* MV and TV prolapse
* Aortic root dilatation
* Aortic dissection
* Dilatation of sinus of Valsalva
* Endocarditis.

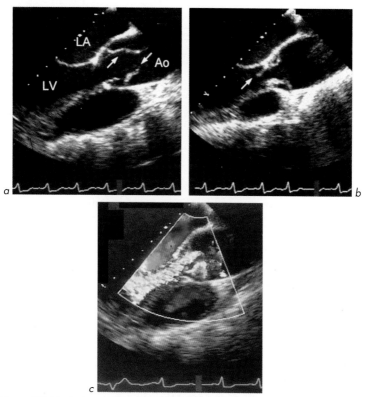

Figure 7.2 Marfan's syndrome. Dissecting aneurysm of ascending aorta. TOE study (aortic long-axis views). **(a)** The dissection flaps are seen (arrows). **(b)** There is prolapse of an aortic valve cusp (arrow). **(c)** Severe aortic regurgitation.

Systemic lupus erythematosus (SLE)

- Pericarditis and effusion
- Infective endocarditis
- Non-infective endocarditis (Libman–Sacks).

Rheumatoid arthritis

- Pericarditis and effusion, occasionally constriction
- Infiltration of rheumatoid nodules, valvular involvement causing regurgitation (aortic > mitral) (rare).

Ankylosing spondylitis

- Aortic root dilatation
- AV thickening
- AR
- Myocardial involvement.

Rheumatic heart disease

Acute rheumatic fever is very rare in Western countries but still common in low-income countries.
- Myocarditis
- Endocarditis (valvulitis)
- Pericarditis
- Consequences – rheumatic valve disease years later.

3. ENDOCRINE

Diabetes

- Effects of co-existent coronary artery disease or hypertension
- LV dysfunction – mild to severe, systolic (like dilated cardiomyopathy) or diastolic (of the 'restrictive type'), often in combination.

Acromegaly

- LVH, particularly of septum
- Dilated LV
- LV dysfunction
- Effects of co-existent coronary artery disease.

Hypothyroidism

- LVH
- LV or RV dilatation and systolic dysfunction, improve with treatment
- Pericardial effusion.

Hyperparathyroidism

- Valvular calcification related to hypercalcaemia – may lead rarely to stenosis or regurgitation.

4. INFILTRATIONS

Amyloid (Fig. 4.9)

- LVH (concentric with a sparkling 'ground glass' appearance)
- Normal LV cavity until late in disease (when dilatation may occur)
- RV hypertrophy
- Hypertrophy of IAS
- Valvular thickening
- Dilated LA and RA
- LV diastolic dysfunction if advanced ('restrictive' mitral flow pattern with very high E-wave and a small A-wave)
- LV systolic dysfunction in advanced cases (poor prognosis)
- Pericardial effusion.

Sarcoid

- Bright IVS with normal or increased thickness and regions of thinning (scarring), especially at base of septum
- Involvement of papillary muscles
- Myocarditis
- Restrictive cardiomyopathy
- LV dilated with abnormal wall motion
- RV involvement
- LA dilatation
- MR and/or TR
- Diastolic or systolic impairment.

Haemochromatosis

In this condition, there is deposition of iron in many organs of the body. Idiopathic haemochromatosis is an autosomal recessive condition. The heart is involved in most advanced cases and the echo features are:

- Dilated cardiomyopathy pattern – dilated LV with reduced systolic function
- Infiltrative pattern (similar to amyloid) – LVH and abnormal myocardial texture.

5. CHRONIC ANAEMIA (INCLUDING HAEMOGLOBINOPATHIES)

- LVH, usually eccentric
- LV dilatation
- LV diastolic dysfunction.

6. HYPERTENSION

- LVH – may show regression on serial echo with treatment
- LV impairment
- Aortic dilatation
- Aortic dissection
- Effects of associated coronary artery disease.

7. RENAL FAILURE

- Pericardial effusion (uraemia)
- LV dysfunction (may improve with haemodialysis)
- Effects of co-existent coronary artery disease.

8. OBESITY

- This is associated with other cardiovascular risks and there may be echo features of hypertensive changes with LVH, changes related to coronary artery disease and diabetes mellitus
- Morbid obesity – this is associated with a high-output state and, in extreme forms, with congestive heart failure
- Lesser degrees of obesity are associated with a slight increase in LV mass and internal dimensions and subtle systolic and diastolic dysfunction but usually there is a weak relationship when corrected for height and lean body mass.

9. MUSCULAR DYSTROPHIES, DYSTROPHIA MYOTONICA, REFSUM'S DISEASE AND FRIEDREICH'S ATAXIA

These genetic neuromuscular abnormalities can have cardiac effects. The echo features are of cardiomyopathies:

- Cardiac involvement typically mimics HCM or dilated cardiomyopathy
- There may be regional variations in LV dysfunction
- Duchenne muscular dystrophy and dystrophia myotonica – autosomal dominant conditions associated with cardiomyopathy
- Refsum's disease (increased plasma phytanic acid due to defective lipid α-oxidase) is associated with a cardiomyopathy
- Friedreich's ataxia (spinocerebellar degeneration, usually autosomal recessive) – the typical echo feature is a posterior LV wall motion abnormality.

10. DIET DRUG VALVULOPATHIES

Treatment with centrally acting appetite suppressant (anorexic) drugs (especially a combination of fenfluramine and phentermine but also dexfenfluramine) has been associated with an unusual form of valve disease. This occurs in 3–15% of cases. The likelihood relates to the duration of treatment and is more likely to happen if the treatment is carried on for more than 6 months, although this is controversial. There are no universally agreed echo findings, and the changes may regress with time if treatment is discontinued. The echo features are:

• MV is most likely to be affected by a lesion. In advanced cases, the valve and chordae are encased in a matrix similar to that seen in carcinoid. This leads to MR. TV is spared
• AR may occur but the echo appearances of the AV are normal
• PHT may occur rarely.

7.9 INDIVIDUALS WITH CANCER

In some societies, cancer affects approximately 1 in 3 (37.8%) women and 2 in 5 (43.3%) men during their lifetime (data from American Cancer Society, 2014). Treatment has improved the quality and length of life for many people with cancer. Many cancers are now cured, with modern chemotherapy, immunotherapy, radiotherapy and surgery.

An integrated approach between oncologists and cardiologists has become essential to the management of many undergoing treatment for cancer. Many centres have developed specialized cardio-oncology clinics.

Echo plays an essential role in the assessment, monitoring and follow-up of the large number of patients undergoing cancer treatment. It is worthwhile exploring the role of echo in some detail.

Echo can assess the presence and effects of the malignancy (e.g. secondary metastatic deposits, pericardial effusion) and of treatment. Echo is widely available, repeatable, versatile, lacks radiation exposure and is safe in patients with co-existing renal disease. In addition to the evaluation of LV and RV size, systolic and diastolic function at rest and during stress, echo allows a comprehensive evaluation of valves, aorta and pericardium. Each patient can act as their own control during treatment.

Echo is helpful in people undergoing treatment with chemotherapy and radiotherapy and has become more relevant with the introduction of newer agents, such as monoclonal antibodies and kinase inhibitors. Many cancers, such as breast and lung, are treated with a combination of agents, either concurrently or sequentially. This can impact upon cardiac function, as can radiotherapy.

CANCER THERAPY-RELATED CARDIAC DYSFUNCTION (CTRCD)

Cancer drugs may cause CTRCD (see Box 7.2). This has been known since the introduction of anthracyclines in the 1960s. Heart failure associated with treatment was recognized as an important adverse effect. As a result, physicians learned to limit the doses used. Several methods have been used to assess CTRCD (e.g. endomyocardial biopsies and monitoring of LVEF). Biopsies are sensitive and specific for identifying anthracycline-induced LV dysfunction. The use of biopsies has diminished. They are invasive, cumulative drug dosages have reduced and non-invasive imaging has improved.

Evaluation of LVEF became widely used to monitor changes in cardiac function, during and after potentially cardiotoxic cancer treatment. The timing of LV dysfunction can vary amongst agents. With anthracyclines, damage occurs immediately after exposure. With other drugs, the time between administration and cardiac dysfunction is more variable. The heart has significant reserve. Alterations in systolic or diastolic parameters may not be overt until a substantial amount of reserve has been exhausted. Cardiac damage may not become apparent until years after receiving cardiotoxic treatment. This is particularly applicable to adult survivors of childhood cancers.

Not all cancer treatments affect the heart in the same way. CTRCD can be classified on the basis of the mechanisms of

---

Box 7.2 CTRCD

- Different definitions of CTRCD have been used
- One definition is a decrease in the LVEF of >10%, to a value of LVEF <53%
- This decrease should be confirmed by repeat echo, 2–3 weeks after the echo showing the initial decrease in LVEF
- LVEF decrease may be further categorized as:
  - ○ Symptomatic (causing heart failure) or asymptomatic
  - ○ Reversible or irreversible:
    - – Reversible (LVEF returns to within 5% of baseline)
    - – Partially reversible (LVEF improved by at least 10%, but remaining >5% below baseline)
    - – Irreversible (remaining within 10% of the nadir), or
    - – Indeterminate (patient not available for re-evaluation)

toxicity of the agents. This can help determine the timing of echo assessments.

Types of drug toxicity

Type I CTRCD

- Characterized by anthracyclines (e.g. doxorubicin)
- Dose-dependent, leads to cell death (apoptosis), therefore irreversible at the cell level
- Early detection and prompt treatment may prevent LV remodelling and progression to heart failure.

Doxorubicin is believed to cause cardiac dysfunction through the generation of reactive oxygen species. The damage to cardiomyocytes is cumulative. The expression of damage relates to pre-existing disease, the state of cardiac reserve at the time of administration, co-existing damage, and individual (including genetic) variability. Once myocytes undergo apoptosis, there is minimal potential for replacement via regeneration. Cardiac damage at the cellular level may be irreversible, but cardiac function may be preserved and compensation optimized through anti-remodelling drug therapy, and/or, less frequently, mechanical intervention. Type I CTRCD drugs have increased potential for long-term cardiac dysfunction, increased morbidity and mortality.

Type II CTRCD

- Characterized by trastuzumab
- Not dose-dependent, does not lead to apoptosis by itself, often reversible.

Trastuzumab (trade names Herceptin® and Herclon®) is a monoclonal antibody binding to human epidermal growth factor receptor 2 (HER2). It is often used in the treatment of HER2-positive breast cancer. This, and several other agents, can cause cardiac dysfunction. They do not seem directly to cause irreversible cell damage in a cumulative dose-dependent manner. Recovery of myocardial function is frequently (but not invariably) seen after their interruption.

Newer cancer drugs include the small-molecule protein kinase inhibitors. It is difficult to generalize about these. They often have different kinase targets. The most problematic agents appear to be those targeting vascular endothelial growth factor (VEGF) and VEGF receptors. These typically are associated with hypertension and ischaemic events. The development of CTRCD may be related to transient impairment of cellular contractile elements or to increased afterload on a compromised ventricle.

The most concerning are the non-selective agents, including sunitinib and sorafenib. Some drugs can target up to 50 different kinases, in addition to the intended target. Because these 'off-target' kinases play important roles in the heart and vasculature, the risk for toxicity is increased. As a result of the non-specific and unpredictable nature of myocardial damage, it is difficult to provide definitive recommendations for monitoring patients receiving these agents.

The role of cardiac assessment and echo in patients receiving cancer drugs is complicated by the fact that type I (doxorubicin) and type II (trastuzumab) agents are often given sequentially or concurrently (see Table 7.5). This may increase cell death indirectly by compromising the environment of marginally compensated cells, contributing to the concern that type II agents can still result in cell death.

Table 7.5 Characteristics of type I and II CTRCD

	Type I drug	Type II drug
Characteristic drug	Doxorubicin	Trastuzumab (Herceptin®, Herclon®)
Clinical course and response to anti-remodelling therapy (e.g. β-blockers, ACE inhibitors)	May stabilize, but underlying damage appears to be permanent and irreversible. Recurrence in months or years may be related to sequential cardiac stress	High likelihood of recovery (to or near baseline cardiac status) in 2–4 months after interruption (reversible)
Dose effects	Cumulative, dose-related	Not dose-related
Effect of rechallenge	High probability of recurrent progressive dysfunction. May result in intractable heart failure or death	Increasing evidence for relative safety of rechallenge (more data needed)

Type I drug examples (e.g. anthracyclines): doxorubicin, daunorubicin, epirubicin, idarubicin and mitoxantrone.

Type II drug examples (e.g. monoclonal antibodies, kinase inhibitors, proteasome inhibitors): trastuzumab, lapatinib, pertuzumab, imatinib, sorafenib, sunitinib, bevacizumab and bortezomib.

Based upon ASE/EACVI guidance 2014.
Plana JC, Galderisi M, Barac A, et al. Expert consensus for multimodality imaging evaluation of adult patients during and after cancer therapy: a report from the American Society of Echocardiography and the European Association of Cardiovascular Imaging. J Am Soc Echocardiogr. 2014;27:911–939.

CLINICAL AND ECHO ASSESSMENT AND MONITORING

Co-operation between oncologists and cardiologists before, during and after cancer treatment is vital. Ideally, a pretreatment cardiac assessment should be performed for every patient due to receive a potentially cardiotoxic agent. This may help cardiologists advise oncologists regarding anticipated risks. If not possible in all patients, it is recommended to perform a baseline cardiac assessment in people considered at high risk for development of CTRCD, such as individuals:

- With a history or clinical findings suggestive of LV systolic dysfunction (e.g. known cardiac ischaemic or non-ischaemic insult)
- At high risk for cardiac events on the basis of risk factors (hypertension, diabetes, hyperlipidaemia, smoking, family history of premature coronary artery disease, age, gender)
- With established cardiovascular disease
- >65 years of age
- Scheduled to receive high doses of type I agents (>350 mg/m^2) or combination chemotherapy with both type I and type II agents.

The baseline and follow-up cardiac assessments (Box 7.3), in addition to a thorough medical history and physical examination, should include:

- ECG to evaluate cardiac rhythm and detect abnormalities (e.g. evidence of previous infarction)
- Cardiac imaging – usually echo – for the evaluation of cardiac structure and function as well as assessment of subclinical LV dysfunction (e.g. by LVEF or reduction in LV systolic function detected by assessment of myocardial mechanics, such as strain analysis – see below)
- Measurement of blood biomarkers such as troponin I (TnI) (see below).

Treatment of subclinical LV dysfunction is based on a strategy of early detection of myocardial disease with imaging and/or biomarkers. This approach may potentially benefit any patient and those without dysfunction are not affected by inappropriate treatment (e.g. unnecessary changes to chemotherapy regimen). The disadvantages are that screening has to be sufficiently accurate to aim to identify all at-risk patients and some patients may have progressed to sufficient damage that treatment may provide only a partial response.

Although combination regimens for heart failure therapy have been reported to be effective, heart failure due to CTRCD is often resistant to therapy if diagnosed late. Therefore, efforts are directed at heart failure prevention.

> **Box 7.3** Cardiac assessment of patients with cancer before, during and after treatment
>
> * Close collaboration between oncologists and cardiologists
> * Careful history and examination
> * Serial ECGs
> * Serial echo studies – full echo assessments, including evidence of subclinical LV dysfunction
> * Serial measurements of biomarkers (e.g. TnI)
> * Consider other imaging modalities (e.g. MUGA scan, cardiac MRI)
> * Timing and frequency of assessments based upon patient's clinical state (risk factors, symptoms, signs) and cancer drug regimen used
> * Consideration whether to continue, discontinue or alter cancer drug regimen
> * Consideration of use of cardioprotective drugs (e.g. β-blockers, angiotensin receptor antagonists)
> * If the LVEF is <53%, there is subclinical LV dysfunction (e.g. GLS – see below – is under the limit of normal or has decreased by >15%), and/or troponins are elevated, there should be discussion between the oncologist and cardiologist of the risk/benefit ratio, and cancer treatment decided at the discretion of the oncologist.

Cardiac and echo baseline and follow-up assessment is recommended (see Box 7.4) on the basis of the specific type of anti-cancer agent received (note that regimens may utilize type I and type II drugs, combined or consecutively).

ECHO EVALUATION OF CARDIAC STRUCTURE AND FUNCTION IN INDIVIDUALS WITH CANCER

LV systolic function

* Echo is suitable for serial evaluation of LV structure and function (see Box 7.5). LVEF should be calculated with the best echo method available (2-D or ideally 3-D echo), combined, if possible, with more specialized techniques (see below)
* With 2-D echo, Simpson's method (Chapter 4) is the technique of choice
* Historically, fractional shortening (FS) using linear measurements from M-mode echo or 2-D echo was used as an LVEF surrogate, to evaluate people with cancer (especially children). This is not ideal. It considers only 2 LV walls (septum and posterior wall) to estimate LVEF. The common occurrence of coronary artery disease in

Box 7.4 Echo timing during cancer drug therapy

Type I drugs

Patients receiving doxorubicin should have:
* A baseline (pre-treatment) echo
* Follow-up echo at the completion of therapy for regimens including doses <240 mg/m^2
* After exceeding the dose of 240 mg/m^2, an evaluation before each additional cycle is necessary.

Type II drugs

Patients receiving trastuzumab should have:
* A baseline (pre-treatment) echo
* Follow-up echo every 3 months during therapy.

Patients receiving the multi-target tyrosine kinase inhibitors (e.g. sunitinib, sorafenib) should have:
* A baseline (pre-treatment) echo
* Follow-up echo at 1 month and
* Follow-up echo every 3 months during therapy.

* Cumulative doses of anthracyclines >400 mg/m^2 previously caused concern, because of an associated 5% risk of heart failure. However, the risk of doxorubicin-related CTRCD is a continuum from 0.2% to 100%, for cumulative doses of 150 to 850 mg/m^2, respectively. The earliest step-up in cardiac events occurs from 250 to 350 mg/m^2 (9% to 18%). Patients who have received doses of anthracyclines <375 mg/m^2 have a rate of subclinical LV dysfunction (LVEF < 50%) of 26% at 6 months after therapy
* If a drug is continued on clinical grounds despite LV functional changes, **reassessment should be undertaken by imaging, ideally echo, and/or troponin, before each additional cycle.** The risk for cardiac events increases with further exposure. Patients' understanding of the risk/benefit analysis should be documented
* In the absence of factors that modify risk to the patient (concomitant risk factors or radiotherapy), **if the echo has been stable during chemotherapy and is normal at 6 months' follow-up** after therapy completion with a type I agent, or troponins have remained negative throughout therapy, additional imaging surveillance for CTRCD is not warranted

Continued

Box 7.4 Echo timing during cancer drug therapy—cont'd

- In the absence of CTRCD or subclinical LV dysfunction with chemotherapy, patients who have received concomitant radiotherapy need to be followed according to published guidelines (e.g. EACVI/ASE expert consensus, see below)
- After completing therapy, especially in patients who were not followed using a strategy of early detection of subclinical LV dysfunction, there should be **a yearly clinical cardiovascular assessment (with echo if appropriate)** looking for symptoms and signs of cardiovascular disease.

Based upon ASE/EACI guidance 2014. Plana JC, Galderisi M, Barac A, et al. Expert consensus for multimodality imaging evaluation of adult patients during and after cancer therapy: a report from the American Society of Echocardiography and the European Association of Cardiovascular Imaging. J Am Soc Echocardiogr. 2014;27:911–939.

patients with cancer and the observation that CTRCD may be regional makes necessary volumetric calculation of LVEF

- LVEF by 2-D echo is a good predictor of cardiac outcomes in the general population, but it has low sensitivity to detect small changes in LV function. For this reason, additional echo assessment of myocardial strain (more sensitive than LVEF) is clinically useful in people with cancer
- Strain is a dimensionless measure of myocardial deformation, which gives an assessment of myocardial mechanics (see also Section 4.7 on long-axis function and Section 4.9 on assessment of dyssynchrony). Strain is the fractional or percentage change in an object's dimension compared to its original dimension. Strain rate is the speed at which deformation occurs
- Strain information can be obtained using either tissue Doppler imaging (TDI) or 2-D echo, using speckle tracking echo (STE)
- STE analyzes the motion of myocardial tissue. On 2-D echo, the myocardium has a speckled appearance on grey-scale images. The movement of these reflections ('speckles') can be tracked by echo machine software and resolved into angle-independent 2-D and 3-D strain-based sequences. These provide quantitative and qualitative information regarding tissue deformation and motion
- STE is increasingly used. Strain results from STE have been validated using MRI. Results correlate with TDI-derived measurements

---

Box 7.5 Importance of echo detection of subclinical LV dysfunction in cancer

- Decreased LVEF at baseline or after anthracyclines is associated with higher rates of cardiac events at follow-up
- Early decreases in radial and longitudinal strain and strain rate were noted using TDI and STE in patients treated with anthracyclines (and in some studies with trastuzumab and taxanes), with or without later decreases in LVEF
- The ideal strategy to detect subclinical LV dysfunction is to compare the GLS measurements during chemotherapy with baseline GLS, with the patient as their own control
- A reduction in GLS of >15% is very likely to be abnormal. A change of <8% appears not to be clinically significant
- The abnormal GLS value should be confirmed by a repeat echo, which should be performed 2–3 weeks after the initial abnormal study
- When examining LVEF and GLS values, keep in mind the load dependency of these measurements. Note the timing of the echo study with respect to intravenous infusion of chemotherapeutic agents (number of days before or after treatment) as well as vital signs during the test (BP and heart rate). Changes in load conditions are frequent and may affect GLS (e.g. volume expansion due to intravenous drugs or volume contraction due to vomiting or diarrhoea)
- If abnormal GLS and/or elevated TnI, discussion between the cardiologist and oncologist as to whether to continue the agent, alter the regimen (at the discretion of the oncologist) and/or consider the initiation of cardioprotective drugs.

- STE advantages over TDI: easier data acquisition; lack of angle dependence; direct strain measurement; multiple simultaneous measurements; ability to perform post-acquisition processing
- A parameter known as global longitudinal strain (GLS) is considered the best measure for the early detection of subclinical LV dysfunction (Fig. 7.3). Ideally, the measurements during chemotherapy should be compared with the baseline value
- Normal values of GLS are approximately −20% to −25% (note negative values). GLS is affected by factors such as age, gender and echo machine used (the same vendor-specific machine should be used in serial studies)
- STE has overcome some of the limitations of TDI. TDI is angle-dependent (requires parallel orientation between direction of motion and ultrasound beam). There is also intra-observer and

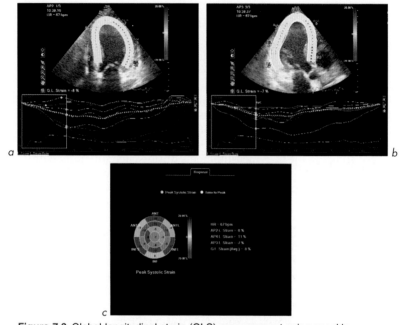

Figure 7.3 Global longitudinal strain (GLS) measurement using speckle tracking echo (STE), in a person with HCM. **(a)** Apical 4-chamber view. **(b)** Apical long-axis view. **(c)** 17-segment LV model. Average GLS = –8%. This is abnormal and is consistent with clinical or subclinical LV dysfunction. Normal values of GLS are approximately –20% to –25% (note negative values).

inter-observer variability and noise interference. TDI allows better time definition and can be also used in case of poor echo windows

- When strain measures are not available to combine with LVEF, LV longitudinal function can be quantified using MV annulus displacement by M-mode echo (MAPSE, see long-axis function, Section 4.7), and/or peak systolic velocity (S_m or s′, S′) at the mitral annulus by pulsed wave TDI.

LV diastolic function

- Conventional assessment and grading of LV diastolic function and non-invasive estimation of LV filling pressures should be performed
- Alterations in LV diastolic function (e.g. as evaluated by Doppler indices of MV flow and E_m [e′] by pulsed TDI) precede alterations in systolic function but the present evidence does not support the role of these indices for predicting later CTRCD.

RV function and PA pressure

• Although prognostic value of RV dysfunction has not been demonstrated in patients undergoing chemotherapy, a quantitative assessment of RV size and function should be performed due to possible RV involvement

• RV abnormalities may occur in people with cancer for several reasons: pre-existing RV dysfunction, neoplastic involvement (primary or metastatic) or as a result of the CTRCD

• PA systolic pressure should be measured. This is particularly important in patients treated with dasatinib, a tyrosine kinase inhibitor, as pulmonary hypertension may be a specific complication.

Valvular disease

• Cardiac valves should be carefully evaluated during and after treatment

• Chemotherapeutic agents do not appear directly to affect valves. Abnormalities may manifest for several reasons, including pre-existing valve lesions, concomitant radiotherapy, infection or CTRCD

• Valve abnormalities may occur due to CTRCD. MR may be caused by annular dilation or apical tethering due to LV dysfunction and LV remodelling. TR may occur because of RV dysfunction or PA hypertension due to CTRCD. MR and TR occur late in CTRCD, after significant ventricular dysfunction

• Primary or secondary cardiac tumours may rarely affect valve function by local effects

• Non-bacterial thrombotic (marantic) endocarditis may occur. More common with left-sided valves

• Valve lesions may vary in size from microscopic to large, bulky lesions, leading to impaired valve closure and regurgitation, which is occasionally severe. Significant valve stenosis is infrequent

• Thromboembolism from valve lesions is a greater risk than haemodynamic impact

• Radiotherapy may cause valve disease. The effect of radiotherapy on valvular apparatus is well described. Echo in patients undergoing radiotherapy should be performed according to published guidelines (e.g. European Association of Cardiovascular Imaging [EACVI]/ASE Expert Consensus, 2013) (see below)

• Chemotherapy may cause pancytopenia, with bacteraemia and sepsis, which may lead to infective endocarditis, with vegetations and valve regurgitation. More likely in underlying valve lesions (e.g. MV prolapse or bicuspid AV) or with indwelling central venous catheters.

Pericardial disease

- Pericardial disease can be associated with cardiac metastasis or be a consequence of chemotherapy or radiotherapy
- Pericardial effusion (Figs. 4.25, 4.26) should be quantified
- Echo features of cardiac tamponade should be assessed, particularly in patients with malignant effusions
- Cardiac MRI should be considered in evaluation of primary tumours of the heart with or without compromise of the pericardium, or when the diagnosis of constrictive pericarditis remains uncertain after a careful echo evaluation.

3-D echo

- 3-D echo is the preferred technique for monitoring LV function and detection of CTRCD
- Advantages include better accuracy in detecting LVEF below the lower limit of normal, better reproducibility and lower temporal variability, as compared with 2-D echo
- Cost, availability, high reliance on image quality and need of operator training currently limit wide application of 3-D echo in the oncology setting.

Contrast echo

- Myocardial contrast agents could be potentially useful when endocardial dropout occurs. Contrast may be used when 2 contiguous LV segments are not well visualized on non-contrast apical images. Contrast agents are not recommended in conjunction with 3-D echo in the longitudinal follow-up of cancer patients.

Stress echo

- May help evaluate patients with intermediate or high pre-test probability for coronary artery disease, who will receive regimens that may cause myocardial ischaemia (e.g. fluorouracil, bevacizumab, sorafenib or sunitinib)
- May help in determination of contractile reserve of patients with evidence of CTRCD.

Indwelling lines

- With implanted ports, tunnelled catheters or peripherally inserted central lines, echo may show tip location with respect to the SVC–RA junction, as well as presence of thrombus or vegetations.

Specific echo challenges

• Patients with breast cancer can present specific imaging challenges. The use of 2-D, 3-D echo and strain imaging to obtain images of diagnostic quality may be limited because of mastectomy, radiotherapy or reconstructive breast implants.

BIOMARKERS IN BLOOD (E.G. TROPONINS) IN INDIVIDUALS WITH CANCER

1. Troponin I or T (TnI or TnT)

• Cardiac troponins are the gold-standard biomarkers for the diagnosis of myocardial injury
• Troponins have potential to provide a robust sensitive diagnostic tool for early detection and monitoring of CTRCD
• Minimally invasive, can be repeated without significant risk
• TnI is a sensitive and specific marker for myocardial injury in adults treated with anthracyclines
• TnI elevation identifies patients at risk for the subsequent development of CTRCD
• Patients with TnI elevations during therapy have higher risk for subsequent cardiovascular events
• TnI should be measured before and 24 hours after each chemotherapy cycle
• Troponins have added prognostic value to echo markers of subclinical LV dysfunction such as GLS. If both TnI and GLS are abnormal, the specificity for the prediction of CTRCD increases to 93%, from 73% (if either alone is abnormal). If both are normal, the negative predictive value is 91%.

2. N-terminal pro-brain natriuretic peptide (NT-proBNP)

• NT-proBNP elevation raises concern for increased LA and LV filling pressures due to CTRCD
• Negative predictive value of NT-proBNP may be useful, but, although likely to reflect elevated filling pressures, is less useful in early CTRCD detection.

NON-ECHO IMAGING MODALITIES ARE USEFUL IN INDIVIDUALS WITH CANCER

Radionuclide ventriculography (multi-gated acquisition – MUGA scan)

• Accurate LVEF calculation
• Highly reproducible
• Main limitations are radiation exposure and lack of ability to report on pericardial and valvular disease, RV function.

Cardiac MRI

- Reference standard in evaluation of LV and RV volumes and LVEF
- If echo quality is suboptimal, cardiac MRI is recommended
- Main limitations are availability and cost
- Useful in situations where discontinuation of chemotherapy is being considered, and/or when there is concern regarding echo or MUGA calculation of LVEF
- Useful in follow-up following radiotherapy
- Standard precautions for MRI safety must be followed. This may be relevant in patients with breast cancer. Some tissue expanders used for breast reconstruction after mastectomy have ferromagnetic components.

CARDIOPROTECTIVE TREATMENT IN CANCER

- Small studies suggest a role for initiation of cardioprotective drugs in the setting of subclinical LV dysfunction
- A variety of agents may be helpful in prevention or early treatment of CTRCD: e.g. dexrazoxane (an iron-chelating derivative of EDTA [ethylenediaminetetraacetic acid], which may be cardioprotective in adults undergoing treatment with anthracyclines), β-blockers, ACE inhibitors, angiotensin receptor antagonists and statins
- As yet, there is a lack of conclusive data (randomized controlled clinical trials) supporting this strategy.

RADIATION-INDUCED HEART DISEASE (RIHD)

There is strong evidence that chest radiotherapy can increase the risk of heart disease. This may occur many years after treatment. Modern radiotherapy techniques are likely to reduce the occurrence and severity of RIHD. The effects of radiation on the heart are reduced, by minimizing dosage, targeting and shielding. However, RIHD may increase in cancer survivors who have received old radiotherapy regimens. The risk of LV dysfunction, valvular abnormality and coronary disease remains in patients treated in the 1980s with chest irradiation. Most information about RIHD is based on studies of patients with breast cancer or Hodgkin's lymphoma. RIHD can also be observed in survivors of lung or oesophageal cancer. The prevalence and severity of abnormalities increase considerably over time from 5 to 20 years, making a case for screening, as they are often clinically unrecognized. Guidance has been published (e.g. EACVI/ASE Expert Consensus, 2013).

Factors associated with higher risk for RIHD

- Younger age (<50 years)
- Cardiovascular risk factors or pre-existing cardiovascular diseases (e.g. diabetes mellitus, smoking, obesity, hypertension, hypercholesterolaemia)
- Exposure to high doses of radiation (>30 Gy)
- High dose of radiation fractions (>2 Gy/day)
- Concomitant chemotherapy (especially anthracyclines)
- Anterior or left chest irradiation (Hodgkin's lymphoma > left-sided breast cancer > right-sided breast cancer)
- Absence of shielding.

Echo is essential in the screening, diagnosis and follow-up of RIHD. Clinicians also have other imaging modalities, such as cardiac MRI, CT or single-photon emission computed tomography (SPECT).

Echo can detect and follow up RIHD

Pericardial disease
- Pericardial effusion
- Pericardial constriction.

Myocardial disease
- Myocarditis
- LV systolic dysfunction
- LV diastolic dysfunction
- Myocardial fibrosis.

Myocardial damage is frequent in cancer survivors treated with radiotherapy. Stress echo can be used to check contractile reserve and follow subclinical LV dysfunction. As with CTRCD, LVEF alone is insufficient. STE to measure GLS is more useful.

Valve disease
- Regurgitation
- Stenosis.

In the first 10 years post-radiation, mild left-sided valve regurgitation is frequent. The clinical significance of mild disease is unclear. Progression to severe disease may take many years. Haemodynamically significant (moderate valve disease) is more common >10 years following radiation. Some studies suggested a higher occurrence of valve disease in women than men.

Coronary artery disease (CAD) and vascular disease
Patients with radiation-induced CAD generally present at a younger age than the general population. The time interval for the

development of significant CAD is 5–10 years. Tests of inducible ischaemia, such as stress echo, SPECT and stress MRI, can give evidence of CAD. Image-based stress testing is indicated in irradiated patients who have angina or who develop new resting regional wall-motion abnormalities on follow-up echo. Studies have shown a role for using CT calcium score or angiography for the evaluation of coronary lesions. Radiation can also be associated with calcification and atheroma of ascending and arch aorta ('porcelain aorta'), which can be detected by CT.

Use of echo for RIHD follow-up evaluation

The ideal strategy for RIHD screening is still debated. The magnitude of the risk of RIHD with modern radiotherapy techniques is not yet well defined. Large prospective studies are required to confirm the optimum surveillance of asymptomatic cancer survivors. This will enable targeted follow-up, screening and intervention.

Baseline (before radiotherapy)

• Pre-treatment cardiovascular screening for risk factors and history and examination should be performed in all patients
• **Echo** in all patients.

Follow-up

• **Yearly** history and examination with attention to symptoms and signs of heart disease
• The development of new cardiopulmonary symptoms or physical signs, such as a new murmur, should prompt **echo** and further investigation
• In high-risk asymptomatic patients (see groups as detailed above, e.g. people who underwent anterior or left-side chest irradiation, particularly if treated for Hodgkin's lymphoma or breast cancer), **echo after 5 years**
• In these high-risk patients, the increased risk of coronary events 5–10 years after radiotherapy makes it reasonable also to consider non-invasive stress imaging (e.g. **stress echo**, stress MRI) to screen for obstructive CAD. Stress testing can be planned **at 5 years and then every 5 years** if the first examination does not show inducible ischaemia
• In lower-risk asymptomatic patients, screening **echo 10 years** after treatment appears reasonable given the high likelihood of diagnosing significant cardiac pathology
• In cases where there are no pre-existing cardiac abnormalities, surveillance **echo every 5 years** after the initial 10-year echo following radiation.

PERFORMING AND REPORTING AN ECHO

8.1 PERFORMING AN ECHO

The echo techniques described so far can be combined to allow a comprehensive transthoracic echo examination to be carried out. There is no ideal set routine for this. Each individual may have their own standard method, which should allow a detailed echo assessment and measurements, without missing out important information. Echo is a practical, learned procedure, and practice is essential to improve. Those new to echo are encouraged to carry out studies under the supervision and guidance of more experienced practitioners. It is safe – no harm can come to the echo patient from ultrasound. With practice, the echo sequence will flow naturally and become second nature.

There are many helpful courses for those new to echocardiography and online and multi-media resources are available (such as the training DVDs produced by the American Society of Echocardiography).

Useful protocols and guidelines have been published, nationally and internationally, which give guidance about the minimum dataset required in an adult echo study (e.g. see British Society of Echocardiography Protocols – Minimum Dataset for a Standard Transthoracic Echocardiogram, 2012 – available online at: http://www.bsecho.org/media/71250/tte_ds_sept_2012.pdf).

National and international societies have also produced syllabuses and accreditation and certification examinations in adult and paediatric TTE and TOE and echo in specific settings, such as critical care (e.g. Accreditation of British Society of Echocardiography, European Society of Cardiology, certification by the National Board of Echocardiography in the USA, etc.).

The following is a suggested routine, with some practical tips and advice.

1. PREPARING FOR AND PERFORMING THE ECHO STUDY

- Explain the reasons for the echo to the patient
- Explain that it is safe and painless and obtain their consent
- It should take 30–45 minutes to complete (this should include reporting time)
- The patient's chest should be bare and so ensure their privacy and dignity
- Offer the patient a gown
- Consider having a chaperone present, as appropriate
- The environment should be warm and quiet with no disturbances and the lighting adjusted to allow the echo machine screen to be well seen
- Attach ECG electrodes (to time echo findings to the cardiac cycle on the ECG):
  - red electrode to right shoulder
  - yellow electrode to left shoulder
  - green electrode to right costal margin
- Attach phonocardiogram if required (to record heart sounds and murmurs)
- Sit next to the patient, to their right side, facing the echo machine (Fig. 8.1)

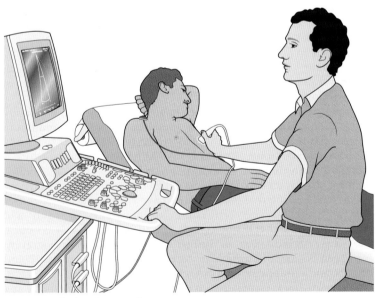

Figure 8.1 Performing an echo.

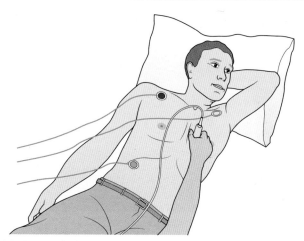

Figure 8.2 Position for left parasternal views.

- Sit upright and ensure that you are comfortable. It is easy to cause back pain if your posture is incorrect, especially after carrying out a number of echo studies in succession!
- Some practitioners may obtain certain echo views (e.g. apical) from the patient's left side. (Some may prefer to carry out the entire study from that side)
- The subject should initially recline at 45° and lie rolled onto their left side (left lateral decubitus position). Their left hand is placed behind their head, their right hand to their right side (Fig. 8.2). You may need to adjust the position of the patient during the study (e.g. roll more to the left, etc.) and for the later views (e.g. subcostal views)
- The echo windows to be used are those in Figure 1.2 and as described in detail below
- Some echo images (e.g. parasternal long-axis) may be better when the patient breathes out and holds. Others (e.g. apical) may be better with a gentle breath held in. Subcostal images may be better with a deep breath held in
- Most practitioners will hold the transducer with their right hand and use the left hand to adjust the echo machine controls to make recordings, etc.
- Place a small volume (~5 mL) of ultrasound gel on the head of the echo transducer. This will allow a fluid interface to allow transmission and reception of ultrasound waves (more effective than passing through air)
- Hold the echo transducer as you would a pen, between the thumb and first 2 fingers (Fig. 8.3)

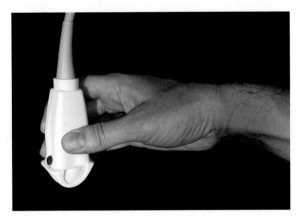

Figure 8.3 Holding an echo transducer.

- Extend your right arm and rest the lower edge of your hand and the transducer perpendicular on the patient's chest wall
- It is important to rest the transducer *lightly* on the chest wall. There is no need to press hard – that may cause unnecessary discomfort to the patient, will squeeze out the echo gel and reduce the fluid interface, and will not improve the echo images
- It will usually only be necessary to make small adjustments to the echo transducer to alter and optimize the echo images
- Eye–hand co-ordination is important. When obtaining and optimizing echo images, resist the temptation to look at your right hand! Make small adjustments to the transducer with your right hand, whilst looking at the echo machine screen
- Note that it may be necessary to adapt the study based upon findings. When performing an echo, do not be afraid or limited from adjusting the transducer position to try to optimize the image
- In each transducer position and echo view, it will be necessary to use the different echo modalities to obtain all the necessary information. A suggested sequence to be used is:
  1. 2-D echo
  2. M-mode echo (particularly useful in parasternal long-axis and subcostal views)
  3. Colour flow mapping Doppler
  4. Pulsed wave Doppler
  5. Continuous wave Doppler
  6. Other echo modalities (e.g. tissue Doppler imaging)
- Some modalities are more useful in particular views. For example, most M-mode measurements of dimensions (e.g. LV systolic and

diastolic dimensions and wall thickness, aortic root diameters, LA diameter, etc.) are made using a parasternal long-axis view. Note that a subcostal view may be a useful alternative if the parasternal views are technically difficult and the images poor. Remember also that the M-mode beam must be perpendicular to the cardiac structures being examined. For continuous wave Doppler, the ultrasound beam should be parallel to the direction of blood flow

- In some views, after obtaining the standard views, it may be helpful to focus on specific parts of the cardiac structures (e.g. after the standard parasternal long-axis view, it may be beneficial to zoom in to the MV and subvalvular apparatus)
- At each echo view, record a small number of cardiac cycles (e.g. 3, or more if patient is in AF).

2. OBTAINING AND OPTIMIZING THE ECHO IMAGES

As with many aspects of echo, this improves with practice and experience (see Box 8.1). Echo is a very practical procedure. Practicing frequently on suitable people will improve skill and eye–hand co-ordination! Remember – echo is safe, as only sound waves are used (no ionizing radiation, etc.). Often, only very small adjustments are needed to improve the echo image.

Images need to be 'on-axis' to allow correct assessment and measurements, for example, cardiac chamber dimensions, function and wall motion (perpendicular for M-mode) and Doppler (parallel to the jet/flow, so velocity is not underestimated). Do not be afraid to adjust the transducer position to obtain better images.

The movements of the transducer (Fig. 8.4) can be:

- Positional – moving the position on the chest wall
- Angulation – tilting – side to side, to left or right or to head (superior) or feet (inferior)
- Rotational – rotating along its long-axis.

In a parasternal long-axis view, for example, the aim is to produce a 2-D echo image where the interventricular septum (IVS) and left ventricular posterior wall (LVPW) are parallel and the IVS and anterior aortic wall are horizontal (at the same height at both sides of the image plane). In most adults, the 3rd intercostal space (ICS) is good, but finding the correct space may involve moving up to the 2nd ICS or down to the 4th ICS. Do not hesitate to explore and to try different transducer positions to obtain better images. This may be necessary as there is anatomical variation between patients (with regards to echo windows, etc.).

There is another helpful rule when trying to optimize images, for example parasternal long-axis views: 'angle for the centre, rotate for the sides'. Imagine the imaging sector divided into 3 equal-sized sectors. In the middle sector, optimize the image (e.g. ensure that MV

Box 8.1 Echo optimization – some technical aspects to consider

- Correct position of patient, e.g. left lateral decubitus for parasternal and apical views, reclining on back at 45° for subcostal and suprasternal views, on right side for right parasternal views
- Correct breathing pattern or breath-holding, e.g. breath out for parasternal, gentle breath in for apical, deep breath in for subcostal views
- Aim for 'on-axis' views, e.g. perpendicular for accurate M-mode measurements and parallel to jet/flow for Doppler measurements
- Frequency of transducer – 3 MHz for most adult studies, giving a resolution of about 0.5 mm
- Ultrasound gel – keep a small volume in the contact area between transducer head and chest wall
- Correct transducer location – position, angle, rotation
- Sector depth – adjust so as much of the whole heart is displayed, with area of interest at centre, unless examining a particular structure when the depth can be adjusted up or down
- Sector size/width – a balance between a wide sector to show a larger area versus a small sector to improve image quality
- Gain – image brightness is adjusted by increasing or decreasing the strength of the ultrasound signal transmitted
- Focus – ultrasound can be focused, by adjusting the sequence in which the crystals in the transducer are activated. Focus just below the area of interest
- Tissue harmonics – settings may be used to improve image quality. In general, higher settings improve quality but increase apparent thickness of highly reflective structures (e.g. valves, pericardium)
- Doppler – colour flow mapping – adjust sector size and location, gain, aliasing velocity
- Doppler – pulsed wave – adjust position of sample volume, baseline, sweep speed
- Doppler – continuous wave – adjust so ultrasound beam is parallel to the jet of interest (remember – it gives maximum velocity at any point along ultrasound beam – does not localize).

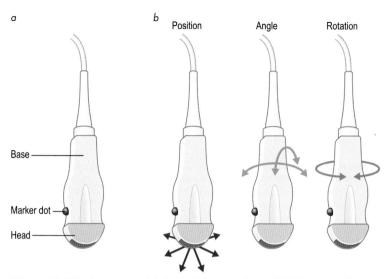

Figure 8.4 Echo transducer. **(a)** Parts of the transducer. **(b)** Movement of the transducer.

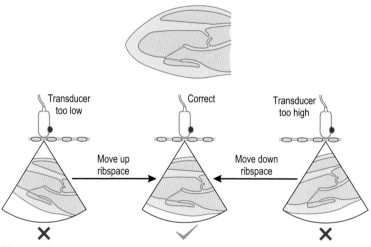

Figure 8.5 Optimizing parasternal long-axis view.

and AV are centred) by angulation of the transducer. When these are optimally positioned, then improve the images in the side sectors by rotation of the transducer on its long-axis.

Figures 8.5 and 8.6 show some aspects of optimizing a parasternal long-axis view and an apical 4-chamber view, respectively. Figure 8.7 shows some other aspects of image optimization.

a **Angulation**

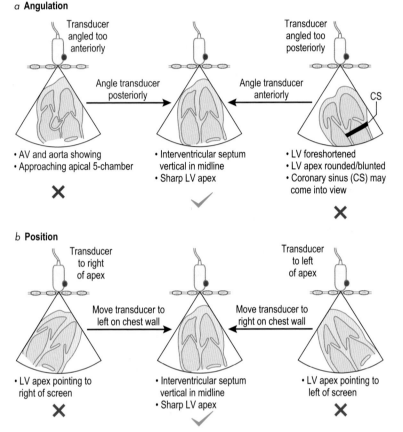

Figure 8.6 Optimizing apical 4-chamber view.

3. ECHO STUDY SEQUENCE (Fig. 8.8)

• 1. Start with parasternal long-axis (PLAX) views
(Fig. 8.8a) – usually up to 3 views

Place the transducer at the left parasternal window (usually the left sternal edge, at the 3rd ICS – not over a rib!). Hold the transducer perpendicular to the chest wall, with the marker on the transducer pointing towards the right shoulder tip.

Use 2-D echo to obtain and optimize an on-axis long-axis view. Figures 8.5 and 8.7 show some advice about image optimization. Use the different echo modalities (as above) and follow the sequence in Figure 8.8a to obtain all the echo information from the PLAX view. By angling the transducer inferiorly and medially (down and in), or superiorly and laterally (up and out), respectively, one can also obtain parasternal RV inflow and RV outflow views (Fig. 8.8a).

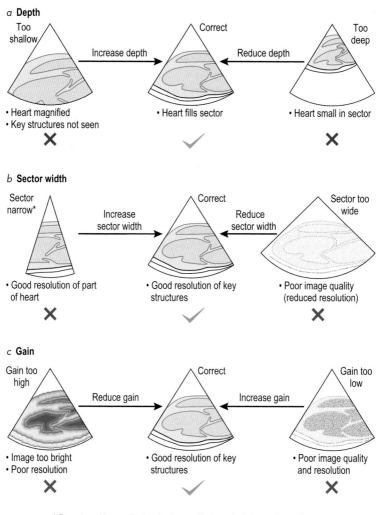

a **Depth**

Too shallow		Correct		Too deep
	Increase depth →		← Reduce depth	

- Heart magnified
- Key structures not seen
✗

- Heart fills sector
✓

- Heart small in sector
✗

b **Sector width**

Sector narrow*		Correct		Sector too wide
	Increase sector width →		← Reduce sector width	

- Good resolution of part of heart
✗

- Good resolution of key structures
✓

- Poor image quality (reduced resolution)
✗

c **Gain**

Gain too high		Correct		Gain too low
	Reduce gain →		← Increase gain	

- Image too bright
- Poor resolution
✗

- Good resolution of key structures
✓

- Poor image quality and resolution
✗

* Parasternal long-axis view is shown. Similar principles apply to other views (e.g. apical 4-chamber, subcostal, etc.)

Figure 8.7 Some aspects of echo image optimization. Parasternal long-axis views are shown. Similar principles apply to other views (e.g. apical 4-chamber, subcostal, etc.). *Note that a narrow sector may be useful in certain circumstances, to focus on particular aspects of cardiac structure. The narrower sector can be angled to one side or another.

- **2. Next, move to the parasternal short-axis (PSAX) views** (Fig. 8.8b) – usually up to 4 views

The transducer is then rotated about 90° clockwise around its long axis to point the marker towards the left shoulder tip, to obtain the PSAX views. In each view, the different echo modalities should be used to obtain the necessary information (Fig. 8.8b). By changing the angulation of the transducer (in an increasingly superior direction), it is possible to obtain echo data at LV apex, papillary muscle, MV level and RV outflow (AV) levels (Fig. 8.8b).

- ## 3. Next, move to obtain the apical views
  (Figs. 8.8c and 8.9) – usually up to 4 views

Apical 4-chamber (A4C) and apical 5-chamber (A5C) views
The transducer is placed at the cardiac apex, with the marker pointing downwards and to the left (Fig. 8.9). It may be necessary to move the position of the transducer on the chest wall or its angulation to obtain an optimized image, with the IVS and IAS running vertically down the mid-line of the screen and without foreshortening of the LV (Figs. 8.6, 8.7). The apical 4-chamber view is obtained. The sequence in Figure 8.8c should be followed to obtain the necessary echo information. By angling the transducer to give a slight upwards (superior) angulation of the echo beam, the apical 5-chamber view is obtained (Fig. 8.8c).

Apical 2-chamber (A2C) and apical long-axis (ALAX, or 3-chamber, A3C) views
For the apical 2-chamber view, the transducer is returned to the apical 4-chamber view position and then rotated approximately 45–60° anticlockwise, so the marker points towards the left shoulder tip. For the apical long-axis (sometimes referred to as 3-chamber) view, the transducer is rotated anticlockwise approximately a further 45–60° from the 2-chamber view (i.e. starting at the standard apical 4-chamber view, the transducer is rotated anticlockwise approximately 90–120°) so it points towards the right shoulder tip. This gives a similar view to the PLAX view, but in a different orientation. Echo measurements are as detailed in Figure 8.8c.

- ## 4. Next, move to the subcostal views
  (Figs. 8.8d and 8.10) – usually 1 or 2 views

The subcostal views are very useful and should be used routinely in every echo study. Many of the parasternal and apical views can be replicated, in a different orientation. It can allow confirmation of previous findings. In some patients (e.g. in an ICU setting), only subcostal views may be technically possible.

The echo subject should be repositioned for the subcostal views. The person lies facing forwards, at 45° (Fig. 8.10). If possible, the person bends the legs up, to relax the abdominal wall muscles. The transducer is placed under the costal margin in the mid-line (under the xiphisternum). The transducer points towards the left shoulder tip, with the marker to the left. The best images are usually obtained with

a **Left parasternal long-axis view: subject in left parasternal position, at 45°**

Tranducer:
• Left sternal edge, 3rd intercostal space
• Marker to right shoulder

1. Parasternal long-axis (PLAX) view

Echo information obtained:

• 2-D: LV (systolic function, regional wall motion), RV, AV, LVOT and diameter, MV, LA, pericardium, pericardial effusion
• M-mode: LVEDD, LVESD, IVSd, IVSs, PWd, PWs, MV, AV, aortic root dimensions, LA dimension
• Colour flow mapping Doppler: AV (AR?), MV (MR?), IVS (VSD?)

(moving the transducer up one intercostal space may allow visualization of the ascending aorta)

2. RV inflow view
(transducer angled inferiorly and medially [down and in] from PLAX)

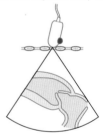

• 2-D: RV, TV, RA
• Colour flow mapping Doppler: TV
• CW Doppler: TV

3. RV outflow view
(transducer angled superiorly and laterally [up and out] from PLAX)

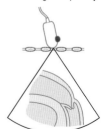

• 2-D: PV, PA, RVOT diameter, PA diameter, left PA
• Colour flow mapping Doppler: RVOT, PV, PA
• PW Doppler: RVOT
• CW Doppler: PV

Figure 8.8 Echo study sequence and information obtained. **(a)** Parasternal long-axis (PLAX) views.   *Continued*

b **Left parasternal short-axis views: subject in left parasternal position, at 45°**

Tranducer:
• Left sternal edge, 3rd intercostal space
• Marker to left shoulder

Echo information obtained:

1. **Parasternal short-axis (PSAX) view–LV papillary muscle level**
(transducer angled inferiorly [down towards feet])*

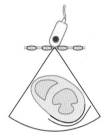

• 2-D: LV , RV, pericardium, pericardial effusion
• M-mode: (if not possible from PLAX) LVEDD, LVESD, IVSd, IVSs, PWd, PWs
• Colour flow mapping Doppler: IVS (VSD?)

(*further inferior angulation shows LV apex)

2. **Parasternal short-axis view–MV level**

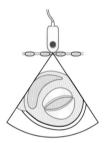

• 2-D: MV (structure, thickness, mobility, calcification, commissural fusion, subvalvar apparatus, vegetations)
• Colour flow mapping Doppler: MV, IVS (VSD?)

3. **Parasternal short-axis view–AV level**
(transducer angled superiorly [up towards head])

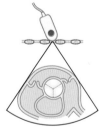

• 2-D: AV, TV, PV, RV, RVOT and diameter, PA and diameter, branch PAs, LA, IAS
• Colour flow mapping Doppler: AV, TV, RVOT, PV, PA, IAS
• PW Doppler: TV, RVOT
• CW Doppler: TV, PV

Figure 8.8, cont'd (b) Parasternal short-axis (PSAX) views. *Continued*

c **Apical views: subject in left parasternal position, at 45°**

Tranducer:
• Apex
• Marker to left axilla

Echo information obtained:

1. **Apical 4-chamber (A4C) view**

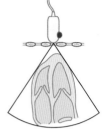

• 2-D: LV (systolic function, regional wall motion, area/ volume in systole and diastole by Simpson's method, LVEF), RV dimensions and area, IVS, MV, TV, LA area/ volume by Simpson's method, RA area, IAS* and mobility, pericardium, pericardial effusion
• M-mode: LV MAPSE, RV TAPSE
• Colour flow mapping Doppler: MV (MR?, vena contracta), TV, IVS (VSD?), IAS (ASD?), pulmonary veins
• PW Doppler: MV, PV, pulmonary veins
• CW Doppler: MV, TV

(*Note – IAS may be poorly seen, as viewed edge-on and 'echo dropout' may give appearance of defect)

• Tissue Doppler imaging: LV lateral and septal mitral annulus, RV lateral tricuspid annulus

2. **Apical 5-chamber (A5C) view**
(transducer angled anteriorly [up towards head] from A4C)

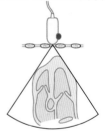

• 2-D: AV, LV, LVOT, LVOT diameter
• Colour flow mapping Doppler: AV (AR?)
• PW Doppler: LVOT
• CW Doppler: AV (V_{max}, VTI)

3. **Apical short-axis (2-chamber, A2C) view**
(marker rotated from A4C view ~45°–60° anticlockwise towards left shoulder)

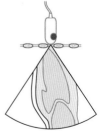

• 2-D: LV (anterior and inferior walls, systolic function, regional wall motion, area/volume in systole and diastole by Simpson's method, LVEF), MV, LA area/volume by Simpson's method, pericardium, pericardial effusion
• Colour flow mapping Doppler: MV
• PW Doppler: MV
• CW Doppler: MV

Figure 8.8, cont'd (c) Apical views.

Continued

Echo information obtained:

4. Apical long-axis (ALAX or 3-chamber, A3C) view
(marker rotated from A4C view ~90°–120° anticlockwise towards right shoulder)

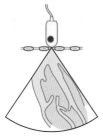

- 2-D: LV, AV, MV, LVOT, LA, pericardium, pericardial effusion
- Colour flow mapping Doppler: MV, LVOT, AV
- PW Doppler: MV, LVOT
- CW Doppler: MV, LVOT, AV

Figure 8.8, cont'd

the person taking in and holding a deep breath. An off-axis 4-chamber view is obtained. By slightly angling the transducer upwards, the AV and LVOT are seen, similar to a 5-chamber view. Rotating the transducer about 90° anticlockwise provides short-axis views through the ventricles and further upwards angulation shows the AV in cross-section and the right-heart structures. Starting from the standard subcostal 4-chamber view, by angling the transducer to the person's right shoulder, the IVC and hepatic veins can be visualized (Fig. 8.8d).

- **5. Next, move to the suprasternal views**
  (Figs. 8.8e and 8.11)

With the patient still reclining at 45°, the head is extended backwards. The transducer is placed in the supraclavicular fossa of the neck, above the sternal notch. The transducer points down, with the marker towards the left shoulder. The aortic arch and descending aorta can be seen, the latter with some leftwards angulation. By angling the transducer to the right, the ascending aorta can be seen. Rotating the transducer about 45° anticlockwise from its initial position gives a short-axis view of the posterior aspect of the LA and the 4 pulmonary veins (this is sometimes termed the 'crab view'). The suprasternal views can be difficult in adults.

- **6. Next, move to the right parasternal views**
  (Figs. 8.8f and 8.12)

These are not routinely performed, but can be helpful in people with AS. The patient rolls to their right side. The transducer is placed in the 2nd or 3rd ICS, with the marker to the left. This allows examination of the ascending aorta and the flow across the AV, for example, for assessing the severity of AS. A dedicated sensitive Doppler transducer with a smaller transducer head (called a PEDOF [*Pulsed Echo DOppler Flow* velocity meter] probe) may be used, but this lacks

d **Subcostal views: subject lying on back, semirecumbant at 45°, knees bent up**

Tranducer:
• Under xiphisternum, angled upwards and to left shoulder
• Marker to left

1. Subcostal 4-chamber (SC4C) view

Echo information obtained:

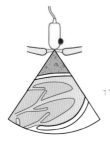

• 2-D: LV (systolic function, regional wall motion), RV, IVS, MV, TV, LA, RA, IAS, pericardium, pericardial effusion
• M-mode: (if not possible from PLAX) LVEDD, LVESD, IVSd, IVSs, PWd, PWs
• Colour flow mapping Doppler: MV (MR?), TV, IVS (VSD?), IAS (ASD?)
• CW Doppler: TV

2. Subcostal inferior vena cava (IVC), hepatic vein and RA (short-axis) view
(transducer angled to subject's right shoulder)

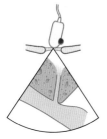

• 2-D: IVC diameter and collapsibillity
• M-mode: IVC diameter and respiratory variation
• PW Doppler: hepatic venous flow

Notes on subcostal echo views:
1. Can be very helpful and should be used routinely. Liver at top of imaging sector.
2. Usually best with subject semirecumbent, knees bent (to relax abdominal wall muscles) with a breath held in.
3. Can be useful in immobile individuals who cannot lie in the left lateral position and in those in an ICU setting.
4. SC4C is similar to an off-axis apical 4-chamber view, rotated by ~90°. Starting at SC4C view:
   • Slight upwards angulation opens the LVOT/AV, giving a view similar to an apical 5-chamber view, from a different orientation.
   • Rotating the transducer anticlockwise by ~90° provides short axis views of LV and RV.
   • Further upwards angulation shows AV in cross-section and right heart (similar to parasternal short-axis views).

Figure 8.8, cont'd (d) Subcostal views.   *Continued*

Echo information obtained:

e **Suprasternal views: subject on back at 45°, neck extended**

Tranducer:
• Above sternal notch, angled down
• Marker to left shoulder

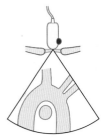

• 2-D: aortic arch anatomy and dimensions
• M-mode: aortic arch diameter
• Colour flow mapping Doppler: aortic arch, coarctation, PDA, right PA
• PW Doppler: descending aorta
• CW Doppler: descending aorta (with imaging transducer or non-imaging Doppler probe [PEDOF]*)

f **Right parasternal views: subject in right lateral position at 45°**
right arm above head, left arm at side

Transducer:
• Right 2nd or 3rd intercostal space, angled down
• Marker to left

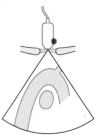

• 2-D: ascending aorta anatomy and dimensions
• CW Doppler: ascending aorta to assess AS (may be measured with non-imaging Doppler probe [PEDOF]*)

Notes on suprasternal and right parasternal echo views:
1. *A non-imaging Doppler probe (PEDOF = Pulsed Echo DOppler Flow velocity meter) may be used.
2. The suprasternal view above shows ascending aorta, arch (with branches: right brachiocephalic [innominate], left common carotid and left subclavian arteries). The right PA is seen under the arch.
3. Right parasternal views may be used to examine the AV and ascending aorta. Other views are possible by altering the position and orientation of the transducer but are not routine in adults. These include right parasternal RVOT, long-axis LVOT and 4-chamber views.

Figure 8.8, cont'd (e) Suprasternal (SSN) view. **(f)** Right parasternal (RPS) view. Notes on SSN and RPS echo views: *A non-imaging Doppler probe (PEDOF) may be used. The SSN view above shows ascending aorta, arch (with branches: right brachiocephalic (innominate), left common carotid and left subclavian arteries). The right PA is seen under the arch. RPS views may be used to examine the AV and ascending aorta. Other views are possible by altering the position and orientation of the transducer but are not routine in adults. These include RPS RVOT, long-axis LVOT and 4-chamber views.

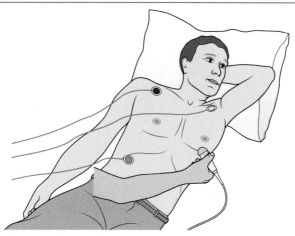

Figure 8.9 Position for apical views.

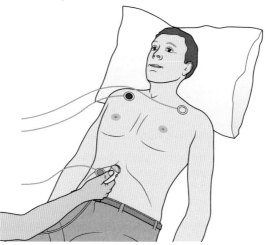

Figure 8.10 Position for subcostal views.

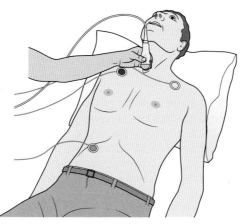

Figure 8.11 Position for suprasternal views.

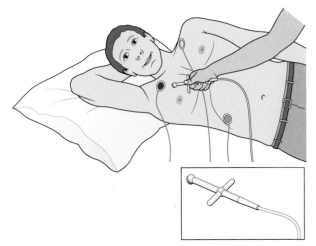

Figure 8.12 Position for right parasternal views. A Doppler only (PEDOF) probe is shown (inset).

2-D echo and colour flow mapping, making positioning of the ultrasound beam more difficult and requiring greater experience and practice. Other echo views are also possible with a standard transducer. Right parasternal views can be difficult in adults.

• 7. The echo study is now complete

Remove the ECG electrodes (and phonocardiogram if used) and allow the patient to remove the ultrasound gel and to dress. The echo information obtained during the study can now be interpreted and used to produce an echo report.

8.2 REPORTING AN ECHO

Having carried out the echo examination, all the information obtained should be analyzed and interpreted.

The images should be reviewed and the necessary measurements and calculations performed. If previous echo studies are available, it may be helpful to review these for comparison. The echo findings should be presented in a report, which can be shared with the requesting individual.

There is no ideal report format, but a standardized report should give all the information in a logical, useful way and an interpretation and conclusion of the findings (Fig. 8.13).

The use of a standardized format ensures that no important information is omitted. A comment should be made regarding the technical quality of the echo study and if it was not possible to obtain any information (e.g. in an adult, it may not be possible to comment on the arch or descending aorta due to poor suprasternal views).

Some report formats group together all the descriptive, anatomical details (e.g. chamber size, and function and valvular anatomy) and have the Doppler studies separately. Other reports integrate all the information together (for each chamber or valve). For example, in a case of severe AS, the report may state: 'Heavily calcified bicuspid AV with restricted opening, valve area 0.4 cm^2 by continuity equation, peak Doppler velocity 4.5 m/s (pressure gradient 81 mmHg) – severe aortic stenosis'.

A suggested echo report format may be based upon the recommendations of the ASE. These published guidelines give an indication of the measurements and descriptive items that should be included in a report.

Cardiology Dept.	**Echocardiography Report**	Page 1 of 2

Name: BROWN, Mary	
MRN: 1234567890	**Study Date: 20/04/2015**
DOB: 07/07/1919	**NHS number: 123456789012**
Age: 95 yrs	**Gender:** Female
	Height, weight: 1.49m , 50kg
Reason For Study: AF new rate controlled on digoxin. BNP 2769 ?cardiac failure	

MMode/2D Measurements & Calculations

RVDd: 4.7 cm	**LVIDd:** 4.1 cm	**FS:** 13.5 %	**LV mass(C)d:** 244.8 grams
IVSd: 1.5 cm	**LVIDs:** 3.5 cm	**EDV(Teich):** 72.1 ml	
	LVPWd: 1.5 cm	**ESV(Teich):** 51.1 ml	
		EF(Teich): 29.2 %	

Ao roTot diam: 2.9 cm	**LVOT diam:** 2.4 cm
Ao root area: 6.7 cm^2	**LVOT area:** 4.6 cm^2
LA dimension: 4.3 cm	

Doppler Measurements & Calculations

MV E max vel: 171.4 cm/sec	**MV V2 max:** 181.0 cm/sec	**Ao V2 max:** 564.0 cm/sec	**LV V1 max PG:** 1.2 mmHg
	MV max PG: 13.1 mmHg	**Ao max PG:** 127.4 mmHg	**LV V1 max: 55.8** cm/sec
	MV V2 mean: 93.6 cm/sec	**Ao V2 mean:** 438.2 cm/sec	
	MV mean PG: 4.5 mmHg	**Ao mean PG:** 83.9 mmHg	
	MV V2 VTI: 35.1 cm	**Ao V2 VTI:** 139.9 cm	
	MVA(VTI): 1.2 cm^2	**AVA(V,D):** 0.45 cm^2	

SV(LVOT): 40.7 ml	**TR max vel:** 314.0 cm/sec	**AS DPI:** 0.06
	TR max PG: 39.4 mmHg	

Left Ventricle
Normal LV size with moderately hypertrophied walls.
Hypokinetic basal-mid septum.
Estimated EF of 25-35%

Severely impaired longitudinal function particularly of the septum.

Right Ventricle
Normal RV size and function.

Atria
The left atrium is mildly dilated. A mass suggestive of myxoma is noted in the left atrium.
Dimensions of the round, smooth LA mass as 2.8 cm, 2.1 cm with area approximately 5.0 cm sq
that appears attached to the interatrial septum. The right atrium is mildly dilated.

Figure 8.13 Echo report.   *Continued*

Mitral Valve
Moderate posterior annular calcification noted. Thickened leaflet tips with some degree of limited excursion. Mildly raised transmitral flow with mean gradient of 4-5 mmHg. Trivial MR.

Tricuspid Valve
Thin and mobile leaflets. RVSP of 39 mmHg + RA pressure. There is moderate tricuspid regurgitation.

Aortic Valve
Severely thickened cusps. Severely raised transaortic flow velocities with peak pressure drop of up to 127 mmHg, mean gradient of 84 mmHg. Trivial AR.

Pulmonic Valve
The pulmonic valve leaflets are thin and pliable; valve motion is normal.

Great Vessels
Normal aortic root dimension. Doppler examination of the descending aorta was normal.

Pericardium/Pleural
There is no pericardial effusion.

Interpretation Summary
Good-fair image quality.   BP: 115/75 mmHg
ECG: AF (78 up to 102 bpm).

Moderate concentric LV hypertrophy with severely reduced LVEF of 25-35%
Severe calcific Aortic Stenosis, trace AR.
Mild mitral stenosis with trace MR.
Left atrial mass suspicious for myxoma.
Raised pulmonary pressure.

___

Finalized By: G.Fielding

Referring Physician: Dr Wilson
Performed By: GF
Figure 8.13, cont'd

Echo report format

The adult echo report should be comprised of the following sections:
1. Patient demographic and other identifying information

2. Echocardiographic evaluation

3. Conclusions and summary.

Each individual echo department can decide the precise format of the echo report, as long as it contains the necessary basic information (see Box 8.2). For example, some laboratories may wish to use a graphic display of LV regional wall motion, whereas other laboratories may choose a text format for reporting this. When possible, the echo information should be coded in database format to facilitate retrieval and communication. Some laboratories include

Box 8.2 **Suggested information to be included in an adult transthoracic echo report**

1. Demographic and other patient identifying information

(1) Patient's name and/or unique identifier (e.g. hospital number), (2) age, (3) gender, (4) indications for test, (5) height, (6) weight, (7) heart rate and rhythm, (8) BP, (9) referring physician, (10) interpreting specialist and (11) date on which study was performed.

Other identifying information which may be helpful includes:
(1) Echo study media location (e.g. disk or tape number); (2) date on which the study was ordered, read, transcribed and verified; (3) location of the patient (e.g. outpatient, inpatient, ICU, etc.); (4) location where study was performed, (5) name or identifying information for person(s) performing the study (e.g. echocardiographer, physician); (6) echo instrument identification; (7) imaging views obtained, or not obtained – especially if the study is suboptimal; (8) additional echo techniques used (e.g. if bubble study or echo contrast agent used).

2. Echocardiographic structural and Doppler evaluation

Cardiac structures
The following cardiac and vascular structures should be commented upon:
1. LV
2. LA
3. RV
4. RA
5. AV
6. MV
7. TV
8. PV
9. Pericardium
10. Aorta
11. PA
12. IVC
13. Pulmonary Veins
14. IVS
15. IAS.

Measurements
Quantitative measurements are preferable (e.g. Doppler velocities). However, qualitative or semi-quantitative assessments are often performed and are frequently adequate.

Continued

Box 8.2 Suggested information to be included in an adult transthoracic echo report—cont'd

The following measurements are commonly included:

1. **LV:**
   a) Size: dimensions or volumes, at end-systole and end-diastole
   b) Wall thickness and/or mass: ventricular septum and LVPW thicknesses (at end-systole and end-diastole) and/or mass (at end-diastole)
   c) Function: assessment of systolic function and regional wall motion. Assessment of diastolic function

2. **LA:**
   Size: area, volume or dimension

3. **Aortic root:**
   Dimensions

4. **Valvular stenosis:**
   a) *For valvular stenosis:* assessment of severity. Measurements that provide an accurate assessment of severity include transvalvular peak and mean gradients and area
   b) *For subvalvular stenosis:* assessment of severity. Measurement of subvalvular gradient provides the most accurate assessment of severity

5. **Valvular regurgitation:**
   Assessment of severity with semi-quantitative descriptive statements and/or quantitative measurements

6. **Prosthetic valves:**
   a) Transvalvular gradient and effective orifice area
   b) Description of regurgitation, if present

7. **Cardiac shunts:**
   Assessment of severity. Measurements of Q_P/Q_S (pulmonary to systemic flow ratio) and/or orifice area or diameter of the defect are often helpful.

Descriptive statements
Describe the echo findings. These comments can be broad in scope. Carefully selected statements should be included in each report, balancing the need for conciseness with completeness, accuracy and detail, in responding to the patient's and referring physician's needs. Echo laboratories may choose to produce brief template statements to construct sentences for use in this section of the report or in the summary.

Continued

Box 8.2 Suggested information to be included in an adult transthoracic echo report—cont'd

3. Conclusions and summary

This section often includes statements that:
1. Answer the question(s) posed by the referring physician
2. Emphasize abnormal findings
3. Compare important differences and similarities of the current study versus previous echo studies, or reports, if available and deemed clinically relevant.

Based upon guidance from www.asecho.org. Gardin JM, Adams DB, Douglas PS, et al. Recommendations for a standardized report for adult transthoracic echocardiography: a report from the American Society of Echocardiography's Nomenclature and Standards Committee and Task Force for a Standardized Echocardiography Report. J Am Soc Echocardiogr. 2002;15:275–290.

some graphical information in the report (e.g. still frames of M-mode, 2-D echo, colour flow mapping images, etc.).

As described above, although there are local variations, it may be ideal, when Doppler descriptive information is included, to integrate this with the corresponding statements derived from echo images. For example, descriptive statements regarding a regurgitant prosthetic AV derived from both echo imaging and Doppler examinations should be grouped together. Some laboratories may prefer to group all the Doppler data in a separate part of the report. This is acceptable as long as all the necessary information is available.

Identification and measurement of some of the structures listed in Box 8.2 may not always be possible or required to provide a comprehensive, clinically relevant echo report. However, it is important for the echo report to include comments on the LV, MV, AV and LA. When images of these structures cannot be recorded or interpreted, the report should state that imaging was suboptimal or impossible. In addition, the indication for a particular echo study may make it crucial to image a particular anatomical structure or to obtain specific Doppler recordings. In this case, it is important for the report to comment on the crucial findings or to note that an adequate recording was not possible.

A sample echocardiogram report is shown in Figure 8.13.

CONCLUSIONS

- Many features of echo are explained by simple physiology
- Echo can give important anatomical and functional information about the heart
- Echo often influences the clinical management of a patient
- Echo is a useful adjunct to the history and examination – *not* an alternative!

FURTHER READING

Abraham W T, Fisher W G, Smith A L et al. Cardiac resynchronization in chronic heart failure. N Engl J Med 2002; 346: 1845–1853

Anand I S, Carson P, Galle E et al. Cardiac resynchronization therapy reduces the risk of hospitalizations in patients with advanced heart failure: results from the Comparison of Medical Therapy, Pacing and Defibrillation in Heart Failure (COMPANION) trial. Circulation 2009; 119: 969–977

Armstrong W F, Ryan T 2010 Feigenbaum's Echocardiography, 7th edn, Lipincott Williams & Wilkins, Philadelphia

Asmi M H, Walsh M J 1998 A Practical Guide to Echocardiography. Hodder Arnold, London

Baumgartner H, Hung J, Bermejo J et al. Echocardiographic assessment of valve stenosis: EAE/ASE recommendations for clinical practice. Eur J Echocardiogr 2009; 10: 1–25

Bax J J, Abraham T, Barold S S, et al. Cardiac resynchronization therapy: part 1 – issues before device implantation. J Am Coll Cardiol 2005; 46: 2153–2167

Bax J J, Abraham T, Barold S S, et al. Cardiac resynchronization therapy: part 2 – issues during and after device implantation and unresolved questions. J Am Coll Cardiol 2005; 46: 2168–2182

Bersten A D, Soni N (eds) 2009 Oh's Intensive Care Manual, 6th edn, Butterworth-Heinemann Elsevier, Oxford

Bristow M R, Saxon L A, Boehmer J et al, for the Comparison of Medical Therapy, Pacing, and Defibrillation in Heart Failure (COMPANION) Investigators. Cardiac-resynchronization therapy with or without an implantable defibrillator in advanced chronic heart failure. N Engl J Med 2004; 350: 2140–2150

Brugada J and Fernández-Armenta J. 2012. ESC E-Journal of Cardiology Practice. Online at: http://www.escardio.org/Guidelines-&-Education/Journals-and-publications/ESC-journals-family/E-journal-of-Cardiology-Practice/Volume-10/Arrhythmogenic-right-ventricular-dyplasia

Chambers J B 1995 Clinical Echocardiography. BMJ Publications, London

Chambers J B 1996 Echocardiography in Primary Care. Parthenon, London

Cheitlin M D, Alpert J S, Armstrong W F et al. ACC/AHA guidelines for the clinical application of echocardiography. Circulation 1997; 95: 1686–1744

Cheitlin M D, Armstrong W F, Aurigemma G P et al. ACC/AHA/ASE 2003 Guideline update for the clinical application of echocardiography: summary article: a report of the American College of Cardiology/American Heart Association Task Force on Practice Guidelines (ACC/AHA/ASE Committee to Update the 1997 Guidelines for the Clinical Application of Echocardiography). Circulation 2003; 108: 1146–1162

Cleland J G F, Daubert J-C, Erdmann E et al. Longer-term effects of cardiac resynchronization therapy on mortality in heart failure [the CArdiac REsynchronization-Heart Failure (CARE-HF) trial extension phase]. Eur Heart J 2006; 16: 1928–1932

Dobb G J 1997 Cardiogenic shock. In: Oh T E (ed) Oh's Intensive Care Manual, 4th edn, Butterworth-Heinemann, Oxford, p 146–152

Eagle K A, Berger P B, Calkins H, et al. ACC/AHA guideline update for perioperative cardiovascular evaluation for noncardiac surgery – executive summary. A report of the American College of Cardiology/American Heart Association Task Force on Practice Guidelines (Committee to update the 1996 guidelines on perioperative cardiovascular evaluation for noncardiac surgery). Circulation 2002; 105: 1257–1267

Everbach E C. Medical diagnostic ultrasound. Physics Today March 2007; 60: 44–48

Focus Issue. Cardiac resynchronization therapy. J Am Coll Cardiol 2005; 46: 2153–2367

Focus on Ultrasound. Physics Today March 2007; 60(3): 1–100

Gardin J M, Adams D B, Douglas P S et al. American Society of Echocardiography recommendations for a standardized report for adult transthoracic echocardiography. J Am Soc Echocardiogr 2002; 15: 275–290. Online at: http://www.asecho.org/wordpress/wp-content/uploads/2013/05/Standardized_Echo_Report_Rev1.pdf

Ghio S, Freemantle N, Scelsi L et al. Long-term left ventricular reverse remodelling with cardiac resynchronization therapy: results from the CARE-HF trial. Eur Heart J 2009; 22: 480–488

Holmberg S 1996 Acute heart failure. In: Julian D G, Camm A J, Fox K M et al (eds) Diseases of the Heart, 2nd edn, W B Saunders, London, p 456–466

Houghton A R 2014 Making Sense of Echocardiography: A Hands-on Guide, 2 edn, CRC Press, Boca Raton

Hung J, Lang R, Flachskampf F, et al 3D echocardiography: a review of the current status and future directions. J Am Soc Echocardiogr 2007; 20: 213–233

Kaddoura S, Oldershaw P J 1994 Pulmonary vascular disease and management of the Eisenmenger reaction. In: Redington A, Shore D, Oldershaw P J (eds) A Practical Guide to Congenital Heart Disease in Adults, W B Saunders, London, p 213–228

Kaddoura S, Poole-Wilson P A 1999 Acute heart failure. In: Dalla Volta S, de Bayes Luna A, Brochier M, et al (eds) Cardiology, McGraw-Hill, Milan, p 517–521

Kaddoura S, Poole-Wilson P A 1999 Cardiogenic shock. In: Dalla Volta S, de Bayes Luna A, Brochier M, et al (eds) Cardiology, McGraw-Hill, Milan, p 535–541

Kaddoura S, Poole-Wilson P A 1999 Chronic heart failure. In: Dalla Volta S, de Bayes Luna A, Brochier M, et al (eds) Cardiology, McGraw-Hill, Milan, p 523–533

Kremkau F W Seeing is believing? Sonographic artefacts. Physics Today March 2007; 60: 84–85

Lancellotti P, Nkomo V T, Badano L P et al. EACVI/ASE Expert Consensus Statement. Expert consensus for multi-modality imaging evaluation of cardiovascular complications of radiotherapy in adults: a report from the European Association of Cardiovascular Imaging and the American Society of Echocardiography. J Am Soc Echocardiogr 2013; 26: 1013–32

Lang R M, Badano L P, Mor-Avi V et al. Recommendations for cardiac chamber quantification by echocardiography in adults: an update from the American Society of Echocardiography and the European Association of Cardiovascular Imaging. J Am Soc Echocardiogr 2015; 28: 1–39

Linde C, Curtis A B, Fonarow G C et al. Cardiac resynchronization therapy in chronic heart failure with moderately reduced left ventricular ejection fraction: lessons from the Multicenter InSync Randomized Clinical Evaluation MIRACLE EF study. Int J Cardiol 2015; 202: 349–355

Mann D L, Zipes D P, Libby P et al. (eds) 2014 Braunwald's Heart Disease. A Textbook of Cardiovascular Medicine, 10th edn, Elsevier Saunders, Philadelphia

Monaghan M J 1990 Practical Echocardiography and Doppler, John Wiley & Sons, Chichester

Mor-Avi V, Lang R, Badano L P et al. Current and evolving echocardiographic techniques for the quantitative evaluation of cardiac mechanics: ASE/EAE consensus statement on methodology and indications. J Am Soc Echocardiogr 2011; 24: 277–313

Moss A J, Hall W J, Cannom D S et al. Cardiac-resynchronization therapy for the prevention of heart-failure events. N Engl J Med 2009; 361: 1329–1338

NICE 2007 NICE technology appraisal guidance 120. Cardiac resynchronization therapy for the treatment of heart failure. Online at: http://www.nice.org.uk/TA120 and updated by NICE 2014 guidance:

NICE 2014 NICE technology appraisal guidance [TA314]. Implantable cardioverter defibrillators and cardiac resynchronisation therapy for arrhythmias and heart failure (review of TA95 and TA120). Online at: http://www.nice.org.uk/guidance/ta314

Otto C M 2012 The Practice of Clinical Echocardiography, 4th edn, Saunders Elsevier, Philadelphia

Otto C M 2013 Textbook of Clinical Echocardiography, 5th edn, Saunders Elsevier, Philadelphia

Otto C M, Schwaegler R G, Freeman R V 2015 Echocardiography Review Guide: Companion to the Textbook of Clinical Echocardiography, 3rd edn, Saunders Elsevier, Philadelphia

Plana J C, Galderisi M, Barac A et al. Expert consensus for multimodality imaging evaluation of adult patients during and after cancer therapy: a report from the American Society of Echocardiography and the European Association of Cardiovascular Imaging. J Am Soc Echocardiogr 2014; 27: 911–939

Regitz-Zagrosek V, Blomström-Lundqvist C, Borghi C et al. ESC Guidelines on the management of cardiovascular diseases during pregnancy. Eur Heart J 2011; 32: 3147–3197

Ruschitzka F, Abraham W T, Singh J P et al. EchoCRT Study Group. Cardiac-resynchronization therapy in heart failure with a narrow QRS complex. N Engl J Med 2013; 369: 1395–1405

Ryding A 2013 Essential Echocardiography, 2nd edn, Churchill Livingstone Elsevier, Edinburgh

St John Sutton M G, Oldershaw P J, Kotler M N (eds) 1996 Textbook of Echocardiography and Doppler in Adults and Children, 2nd edn, Blackwell Science, Cambridge

St John Sutton M G, Plappert T, Abraham W T et al. Multicenter InSync Randomized Clinical Evaluation (MIRACLE) Study Group. Effect of cardiac resynchronization therapy on left ventricular size and function in chronic heart failure. Circulation 2003; 107: 1985–1990

St John Sutton M G, Plappert T, Hilpisch K E et al. Sustained reverse left ventricular structural remodeling with cardiac resynchronization at one year is a function of etiology: quantitative Doppler echocardiographic evidence from the Multicenter InSync Randomized Clinical Evaluation (MIRACLE). Circulation. 2006; 113: 266–72

Sutherland G R, Roelandt J R T C, Fraser A G, Anderson R H 1991 Transoesophageal Echocardiography in Clinical Practice. Gower Medical, London

Swanton R H, Banerjee S 2008 Swanton's Cardiology, 6th edn, Blackwell Publishing, Oxford

Thorne S, MacGregor A, Nelson-Piercy C. Risks of contraception and pregnancy in heart disease. Heart 2006; 92: 1520–1525.

Vardas P E, Auricchio A, Blanc J J et al. European Society of Cardiology 2007 Guidelines for cardiac pacing and cardiac resynchronization therapy: the task force for cardiac resynchronization therapy of the European Society of Cardiology. Eur Heart J 2007; 28: 2256–2295

Wharton G, Steeds R, Rana B et al. BSE protocols. Minimum dataset for a standard transthoracic echocardiogram 2012. Online at: http://www.bsecho.org/media/71250/tte_ds_sept_2012 .pdf

Winter S, Nesser H J 2007 Echocardiography for Cardiac Resynchronization. The Next Step. Handbook Medtronic Europe, Vienna

Young J B, Abraham W T, Smith A L et al. Combined cardiac resynchronization and implantable cardioversion defibrillation in advanced chronic heart failure: the MIRACLE ICD Trial. JAMA 2003; 289: 2685–2694

Yu C-M, Hayes D L. Cardiac resynchronization therapy: state of the art 2013. Eur Heart J 2013; 34: 1396–1403

Zoghbi W A, Enriquez-Sarano M, Foster E et al. Recommendations for evaluation of the severity of native valvular regurgitation with two-dimensional and Doppler echocardiography. J Am Soc Echocardiogr 2003; 16: 777–802

WEBSITES PROVIDING USEFUL INFORMATION, EDUCATION AND GUIDELINES

American College of Cardiology. <http://www.acc.org>.
American Heart Association. <http://www.heart.org/HEARTORG/>.
American Society of Echocardiography. <http://www.asecho.org>.
British Society of Echocardiography. <http://www.bsecho.org>.
European Society of Cardiology. <http://www.escardio.org>.
National Institute for Health and Care Excellence. <http://www.nice.org.uk>.

INDEX

Page numbers followed by "*f*" indicate figures, "*t*" indicate tables, and "*b*" indicate boxes.